Guide to Inpatient Clinical Documentation Improvement

Strategies to Ensure Compliance and Correct Reimbursement

Ruthann Russo, JD, MPH, RHIT

OPUS COMMUNICATIONS
A Division of *hc*Pro

Guide to Inpatient Clinical Documentation Improvement: Strategies to Ensure Compliance and Correct Reimbursement is published by Opus Communications, Inc., a Division of HCPro.

 5 4 3 2 1

ISBN 1-57839-193-8

HCPro provides information resources for the healthcare industry.

HCPro is not affiliated in any way with the Joint Commission on Accreditation of Healthcare Organizations.

Ruthann Russo, JD, MPH, RHIT, Author
Claudia Hoffacker, Group Publisher
John Leonard, Senior Managing Editor
Laura Mackey, Managing Editor
Jean St. Pierre, Creative Director
Mike Mirabello, Senior Graphic Artist
Sandra Wedgwood, Layout Artist
Shane Katz, Cover Designer
Suzanne Perney, Vice President/Publisher

Advice given is general. Readers should consult professional counsel for specific legal, ethical, or clinical questions. Arrangements can be made for quantity discounts.

For more information, contact:

Opus Communications
A Division of HCPro
P.O. Box 1168
Marblehead, MA 01945
Telephone: 800/650-6787 or 781/639-1872
Fax: 781/639-2982
E-mail: customer_service@hcpro.com

Visit Opus Communications at its World Wide Web sites: *www.hcmarketplace.com, www.hcpro.com, www.himinfo.com,* and *www.complianceinfo.com*

Table of Contents

List of Figures

About the Author

Ruthann Russo, JD, MPH, RHIT, is the CEO and principal with HP3 Healthcare Concepts. She is responsible for creating the firm's Clinical Documentation Improvement program and the CDI Toolkit. She provides consulting and does presentations on Reimbursement Strategies for healthcare providers across the nation. She created and produced the Healthcare Reimbursement and Documentation Improvement Video Series. She designed and conducted the National Inpatient and Outpatient Coder Surveys. She is an editor for *JustCoding.com* and has created web-based coder training programs. She has been a product reviewer for the *Journal of Healthcare Compliance*. In addition, she has authored several books including, *Seven Steps to HIM Compliance* and *Coding Compliance: A Practical Guide to the Audit Process,* both published by Opus Communications, a division of HCPro.

Ms. Russo earned her juris doctorate degree from American University and her Master's in Public Health from Robert Wood Johnson Medical School/Rutgers University. She is a doctoral candidate in business at Nova Southeastern University, where she is researching physician attitudes and opinions about documentation.

INTRODUCTION

Introduction

Incomplete documentation in patient medical records can cause inaccurate statistical databases, erroneous financial planning, poor clinical preparation, and lost revenue for healthcare organizations. That's why every organization should ensure accurate and complete clinical documentation—at any cost.

Documentation improvement is not a new concept in healthcare. It joins a number of evolving trends in the U.S. healthcare system, including the following:

- First, the clinical focus has shifted from postponing care until patients are severely ill to providing proactive, preventive medical care. Reflecting this trend, the past decade has seen fewer but more severe inpatient admissions and an increase in outpatient admissions.
- Next, the pace of health information management (HIM) departments in computerizing their medical records continues to increase. The government has responded to this trend by implementing privacy and security protections through the Health Insurance Portability and Accountability Act of 1996 (HIPAA).
- Finally, HIPAA has changed the way healthcare providers receive reimbursement as well. The change began with the Medicare fraud and abuse initiatives of the 1990s. Policy updates from the Centers for Medicare & Medicaid Services (CMS), focusing on physician documentation, continue to affect the reimbursement process.

This book describes the third evolution in health care—documentation and its implications. We focus not only on the components of good patient documentation but also, more important, on ensuring that the provider receives appropriate payment. For its fundamentals, this book relies on current CMS policy, as well as on the guidelines of the American Hospital Association's *Coding Clinic,* which the industry acknowledges as the official source for coding and documentation. The book you see now deals with inpatient documentation. Future updates will focus on various outpatient settings.

We will refer to the following inpatient documentation model, which includes all players in the process, throughout the book:

AMD → **ODC** → **AMD** → **OMD** → **AMD** → **COD** → **AMD** → **BILL**

AMD = attending physician documentation.
ODC = other documentation. This would include all other nonphysician documentation on the patient's record, such as nursing notes, test results, and documentation from other nonphysician clinicians.
OMD = other physicians (other than the attending physician) who are treating the patient. This would include consultants, anesthesiologists, pathologists, and any other physicians documenting in the patient's record.
COD = coder or the final coding that occurs after the patient is discharged
BILL = billing, or the final bill generated for the patient's stay

This model stresses the two most important aspects of patient medical record documentation:

1. The attending physician's documentation is key throughout the patient's stay. In each case, the model stresses the fact that, in good documentation practices, it is important for the attending physician to either interpret the documentation of other clinicians or tests—or, confirm the findings of other physicians.

2. Documentation is the key to appropriate billing. In each case, documentation forms the basis for coding and billing.

We will visit this model throughout the book and describe the various stages represented in the model.

Once we have discussed the origins and importance of documentation in the patient's record, we will describe the necessary components of a program for ensuring excellent clinical documentation. We describe steps that a healthcare organization should take to monitor the extent to which inpatient documentation supports the actual care provided to the patient.

To recap, incomplete documentation can result in inaccurate databases, financial planning, clinical preparation, and gross revenue. Because of these implications, documentation improvement should be a wide-ranging process in every healthcare organization. We discuss who should be involved in such a program and how a program could be organized. We also provide examples of tools that can be used in implementing an effective documentation improvement program. And, finally, we provide tracking and management mechanisms to ensure that a fully implemented program will remain effective.

Use this book as a guide. It lays out a complete documentation improvement program, but every organization is unique. Consider your own organization's philosophies and customs when you implement your own program.

Before we begin, however, a word of caution: The process of documentation review and improvement assumes a high degree of proficiency in coding. If you are not already certain that your coding is of the highest degree of accuracy possible, you will need to focus on improving it. Your organization has to have excellent coding processes in place before you begin documentation improvement.

CHAPTER 1

Clinical Documentation in Patient Records

Clinical Documentation in Patient Records

Why should healthcare organizations care about the clinical documentation in their patient records? With so many competing interests for a healthcare organization's attention today, those topics that get priority need a long list of criteria to justify the organization's attention. We address these criteria below, but first let's look at what constitutes documentation in a patient's record.

What is clinical documentation in a patient's record?

Clinical documentation in a patient's record includes any and all documentation that relates to patient care during a visit, a stay, or an encounter. In the inpatient setting, some of the important pieces of inpatient documentation include the following:

Attending physician documentation

In the acute care inpatient setting, the attending physician bears the primary responsibility for all documentation in the patient's record. The attending physician determines the relevance and importance of all other caregivers' notations in the patient's record. Some of the more important items of clinical documentation by the attending physician during the patient's stay are listed below:

History and physical (H&P)

The H&P is one of the first pieces of documentation that appear on the patient's record. This document usually includes not only information pertaining to the patient's health in the past but also, more important, the present. Here, the attending physician should document his or her assessment of the patient's current state of health. If the attending physician is working with symptoms and differential diagnoses at the time of the H&P exam, he or she should document these symptoms and diagnoses at that time. Although those conditions may be eliminated once a definitive diagnosis has been established, it is important to

Chapter 1

understand and document what the physician was working with in terms of initial or "working" diagnoses. This information may be needed to substantiate any tests or consults that are ordered during the patient's stay.

Making differential diagnoses

EXAMPLE: If a patient is admitted with syncope, and the physician orders both a neurological as well as a cardiology consult, it is important to know that the attending is working with differential diagnoses of "possible CVA" and "arrhythmia." These diagnoses, one neurological and the other cardiological, justify the ordering of a consult from each clinical area.

Progress notes

Progress notes from the attending physician chronicle the entire patient stay. Ideally, the physician should record progress notes on every day of the patient's stay. And in cases where the patient's condition is changing quickly, more frequent progress notes may be warranted. (For a review of the minimum requirements for the frequency of progress notes, see Chapter 2). Progress notes usually contain information regarding changes, if any, in the patient's condition. Any clinician treating the patient can add to the progress notes, but if they are to be used for coding, they must come from the physician. Responses to testing, treatment, and medications should be recorded. More important, the attending physician should document, on an ongoing basis, any new diagnoses. The importance of placing clinical documentation in the progress notes, as opposed to waiting to enter it in the discharge summary, cannot be stressed enough. In addition to chronicling the patient's care, progress notes are also the best place for the attending physician to

- state agreement with a consultant's report
- determine the significance of ancillary test results (i.e., lab, radiology)
- eliminate or add working or differential diagnoses
- state whether a patient has any conditions that should be defined as "possible," "probable," or "rule out"

Orders

The attending physician must provide an order for every episode of treatment and care that the patient receives. Without this direction from the attending physician, the team attending to the patient would be immobilized. It is especially important for the attending physician to document the reason why an order is given. This information justifies in complete detail the actions of the physician in treating the patient's condition.

Procedure reports (for attending surgeons)

A surgeon should dictate reports for all procedures performed during the patient's stay. The surgeon initially records findings at the time of surgery in the progress notes. But a more detailed accounting of the procedure should appear in the dictated operative report. The body of the report should document every possible detail of the procedure.

Documenting the Diagnosis for an Order

EXAMPLE: For an order of antibiotics for a patient, rather than just "Cipro 100mg b.i.d.," it would be more useful for the attending physician to document "Cipro for UTI 100mg b.i.d." Then coders and auditors will know what the Cipro was for.

Discharge summary

The discharge summary is considered the synopsis of all events recorded during the patient's stay. It is important that the discharge summary is just that: a summary of events already chronicled in the patient's record. Events, diagnoses, and assessments should not be recorded for the first time in the patient's discharge summary. At the very least, clinical evidence of every condition documented in the discharge summary should be available in the patient's H&P, progress notes, orders, and operating room reports.

Other physician documentation

In most inpatient cases, other physicians besides the attending physician provide documentation in the patient's record. Consultants, anesthesiologists, and pathologists may contribute to the record of a patient undergoing surgery. Specialists may also include the radiologists and cardiologists responsible for interpreting that patient's diagnostic test results. Let's address those documents individually.

Consultation reports

When a consultant accepts an attending physician's request for a consultation, the consultant is responsible for documenting his or her findings in the patient's record. The consultation report should include the results of any H&P performed independently by the consultant, any test findings, and his or her expert opinion concerning the patient's condition. The consultant may be providing a second opinion, determining the patient's actual diagnosis, or assessing test results. Regardless of the consultant's findings, the attending physician still has the final say about the patient's condition. In the American Hospital Association's (AHA) *Coding Clinic*, the official guide for ICD-9-CM coding, the AHA declares that when there is a disagreement between the attending physician and another physician who's treating an inpatient, the attending physician's opinion always takes precedence. A broad application of this policy would require the attending physician to agree with (or redocument) any findings of the consultant in order for those findings to be considered valid.

Anesthesia reports

In the case of any patient scheduled to undergo surgery, Medicare's Conditions of Participation (COP) require an anesthesiology evaluation both before and after surgery. Before surgery, the anesthesiologist must determine any conditions the patient may have that would require special treatment or management during the surgical episode. Following surgery, the anesthesiologist must clearly document any condition that would impact the patient's care. Again, it is advisable for the attending physician to document his or her agreement with the anesthesiologist's findings if the coders and abstractors are to rely upon the anesthesiologist's documentation. Note that this policy pertains only to the inpatient setting. Currently, in the outpatient setting, it is acceptable to rely upon the anesthesiologist's documentation without validation from the attending physician.

Pathology reports

Tissue removed during a surgical episode is sent to pathology for analysis. The pathologist is responsible for dictating a report that details the findings of the pathological analysis. If the attending physician agrees, this information provides additional detail regarding the patient's condition during the stay.

Radiology/Nuclear medicine reports

If an attending physician orders radiology tests during a patient's stay, a radiologist performs and interprets those tests, dictating his or her findings and assessment in a radiology report. Generally, the radiologist is said to provide an "impression," which is not considered official until the attending physician concurs with the radiologist's assessment.

Cardiology reports

If an attending physician orders an electrocardiogram, echocardiogram, or other cardiology test, a cardiologist performs and interprets the tests. The cardiologist is then responsible for dictating his or her findings and assessment of the results. The impression provided by the cardiologist is not considered to be an official assessment or diagnosis for the patient until the attending physician corroborates it.

Other clinical documentation

Other clinical documentation in the patient's record comes from the nursing staff and other ancillary clinical staff who are treating the patient. The documentation provided by these clinicians is extremely important in providing a complete picture of the patient's stay. From a reimbursement and coding perspective, the documentation these clinicians provide is "supplementary" to the attending physician, but this record is rich in detail that is often lacking in the attending physician's notes. However, unless the attending physician verifies the conditions noted by other clinicians in the patient's record, documentation from other clinical staff may not be relied upon for coding and abstracting purposes. And in the final analysis, all documentation in the patient's record must be coded and abstracted if it is to survive. Once the patient is discharged, the information in the record is relayed to insurance companies, Medicare, cancer registries, research banks, and the like as a result of the coding provided after discharge. So without the attending physician's acknowledgment of the documentation of detail provided by ancillary clinicians, this information becomes forever lost in the patient record.

Why clinical documentation in a patient's record is important

Patient care and quality

The clinical documentation in a patient's record forms the basis for current and future care of that patient by the healthcare provider. Clinicians in the healthcare facility will rely on this record in making decisions regarding the patient's care. This record includes everything from the more "objective" type of documentation, such as the results of laboratory tests, to the more "subjective" type of documentation, such as a consultant's opinion regarding the patient's condition. In either case, the documentation should be as complete and detailed as possible. Unfortunately, most attending physicians have very little time to dedicate to extensive documentation. They prefer to spend their time actually treating the patient, not documenting the treatment. However, it is important to understand that the treatment of the patient includes not only "one-on-one" care, but also an accurate record of that care. And there is no better time to document the care given a patient than when the physician is actually treating the patient. Documentation concurrent with treatment is the best way to accurately record care of the patient. Concurrent documentation is reliable, accurate, and most likely to actually reflect what occurred during the patient encounter. Current and future care is more likely to be of a higher quality when it is based on accurate historical information about the patient.

"Physicians need to validate nursing documentation"

EXAMPLE: A nursing note documents a patient with postoperative urinary retention. The attending physician orders a Foley catheter placed, but does not document the reason for the order. The nursing staff places the catheter and notes that finally, on the second day following the operation, the patient has begun to urinate. In this case, although there is sufficient documentation that the patient had postoperative urinary retention, this condition cannot be coded unless the attending physician confirms it in the patient's record.

Legal protection

Detailed documentation can provide strong legal protection to the healthcare organization. In an action, a court will construe the absence of documentation as evidence against the defendant. Therefore, it is important that the patient's medical record contain detailed, complete, and accurate documentation in the event that the document is needed as evidence in a legal proceeding.

Operations and ongoing management

Healthcare administrators use the data abstracted from a hospital inpatient record in the form of ICD-9-CM diagnostic and procedural codes to plan for operations and ongoing management. For example, the cardiology product line team may be following and trending the abstracted data for all cardiology diagnoses and cardiac catheterizations on a monthly basis. If diagnostic or procedural information is not clearly documented in the patient's record, it cannot be coded and will not appear on the management team's abstract. Without accurate data, effective operational management could be impeded.

Strategic and financial planning

Prospective payment for inpatient cases relies upon ICD-9-CM diagnostic and procedural coding, which relies upon complete and accurate documentation in the patient's record of diagnoses and procedures performed during the stay. Inaccurate documentation results in erroneous coding assignment and, eventually, to imprecise DRG assignment and payment to the hospital. Financial planning and budgeting use prospective payment (DRG assignment) as the basis for gross revenue receipt for inpatient stays. Sloppy documentation can have a significant impact on the hospital budgeting and financial planning process.

Research

Teaching hospitals, state hospital associations, professional medical associations, government entities, and other organizations use coded data in the form of ICD-9-CM codes for research in many clinical areas. Researchers assume that the data is accurate and make projections based upon the data. In the event that poor documentation has resulted in erroneous coded data, the value of such research activities is questionable.

Reimbursement/Gross revenue

One of the most significant effects of incomplete documentation in a patient's medical record is inaccurate reimbursement to the hospital. In the absence of accurate documentation, a hospital should assume that revenues will be inaccurate as well. The model in Figure 1.1 demonstrates the direct relationship between documentation and billing. This model's components show that all the workers in any healthcare organization are involved in the clinical documentation of an inpatient's care.

This model stresses the two most important aspects of patient medical record documentation:

1. The attending physician's documentation is key throughout the patient's stay. The model stresses the fact that in good documentation practices, it is important that the attending physician to interpret the documentation of other clinicians, evaluate test results, and confirm the findings of other physicians.

Figure 1.1 **Model for clinical documentation in the patient's record**

AMD → ODC → AMD → OMD → AMD → COD → AMD → BILL

AMD = Attending physician documentation

ODC = Other documentation (Including all other non-physician documentation in the patient's record like nursing notes, test results, and documentation from other non-physician clinicians

OMD = Other physicians (other than the attending physician) who are treating the patient. This would include consultants, anesthesiologists, pathologists, and any other physicians documenting in the patient's record.

COD = Coder or the final coding that occurs after the patient is discharged

BILL = Billing or the final bill that is generated for the patient's stay

2. Documentation is the key to appropriate billing. In each case, documentation forms the basis for coding and the eventual bill that is generated to represent the charges for the patient's care.

We will revisit this model throughout the book and describe the various stages represented in the model in more detail.

The DRG system and how it works

The clinical documentation model noted above describes the process by which documentation is translated into the bill for the patient's care. To provide additional detail, we will describe the basis of the prospective payment system (PPS) for inpatient reimbursement, also known as diagnosis-related groups (DRGs). Please note that we have simplified the DRG assignment process noted below and limited it primarily to those data that directly impact documentation and coding. There are additional elements that impact DRG assignment, but they are not addressed within this context. See Figure 1.2 for a chart of the flow of information in DRG assignment.

Figure 1.2 **Flow of information in DRG assignment**

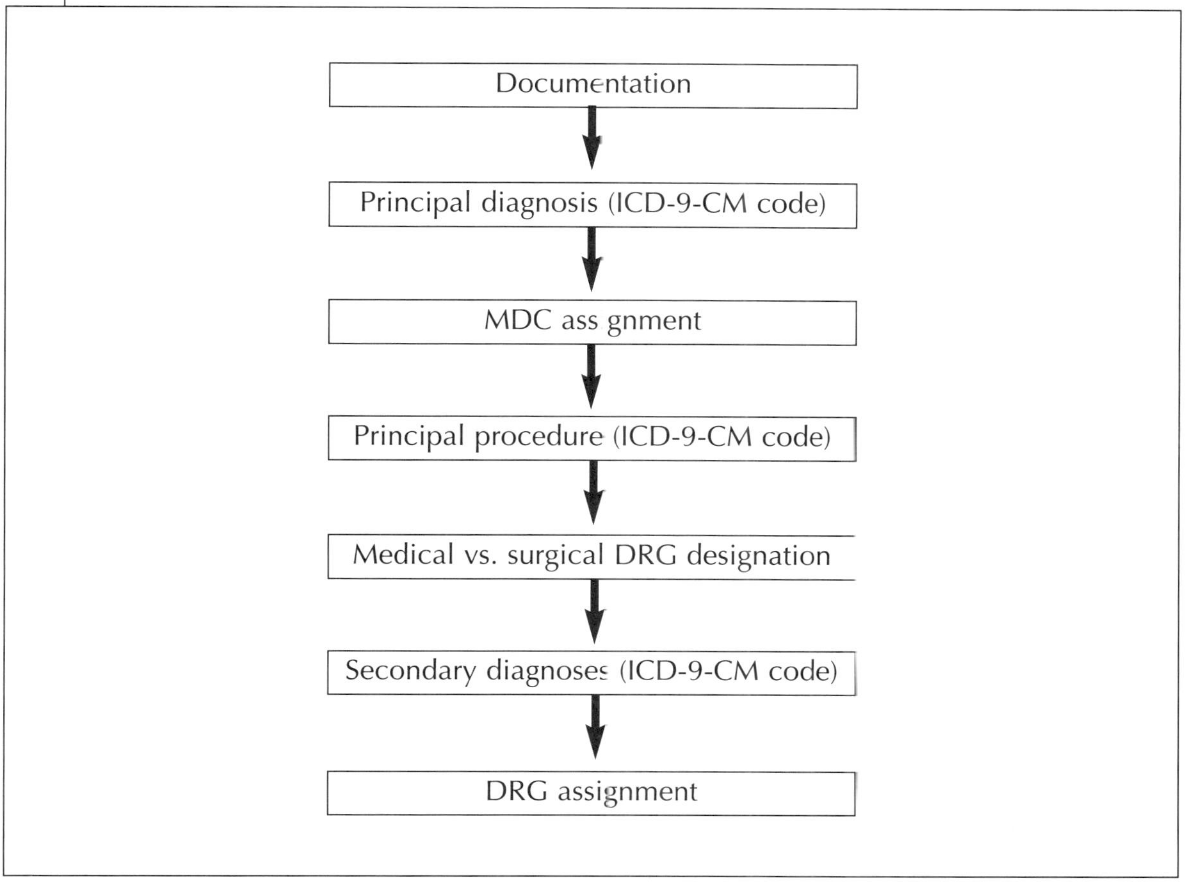

The steps in DRG assignment[1]

Documentation

The first step in DRG assignment for prospective payment is the physician's documentation in the patient's record. In fact, that documentation serves as the basis for all final coding in the inpatient record.

Principal diagnosis code assignment

After discharge, the coder assigns final coding based on documentation in the patient's record. Specifically, the coder "translates" the physician's clinical documentation into ICD-9-CM codes. For the principal diagnosis, the coder must identify "the condition, established after study, to have occasioned the admission of the patient to the hospital." This is the official definition of principal diagnosis, and once it has been identified and coded, the next steps in DRG assignment can proceed.

Major diagnostic category assignment

Based upon principal diagnosis assignment, every case is assigned to a major diagnostic category (MDCs). In general, MDCs are organized around body systems, such as the respiratory system (MDC 4) or the cardiovascular system (MDC 5). See Figure 1.3 for a list of MDCs.

Figure 1.3 **Major Diagnostic Category Listing**

1. Diseases and disorders of the nervous system
2. Diseases and disorders of the eye
3. Diseases and disorders of the ear, nose, mouth and throat
4. Diseases and disorders of the respiratory system
5. Diseases and disorders of the circulatory system
6. Diseases and disorders of the digestive system
7. Diseases and disorders of the hepatobiliary system and pancreas
8. Diseases and disorders of the musculoskeletal system
9. Diseases and disorders of the skin, subcutaneous tissue, and breast
10. Endocrine, nutritional and metabolic diseases and disorders
11. Diseases and disorders of the kidney and urinary tract
12. Diseases and disorders of the male reproductive system
13. Diseases and disorders of the female reproductive system
14. Pregnancy, childbirth, and the puerperium system
15. Newborns and other neonates with conditions originating in the perinatal period
16. Diseases and disorders of the blood, blood forming organs
17. Myeloproliferative diseases and disorders, poorly differentiated neoplasm
18. Infectious and parasitic diseases, systemic or unspecified sites
19. Mental diseases and disorders
20. Alcohol/drug use and alcohol- or drug-induced organic mental disorders
21. Injuries, poisonings, and toxic effects of drugs
22. Burns
23. Factors influencing health status and other contacts with health services
24. Multiple significant trauma
25. Infections caused by the human immunodeficiency virus

Principal procedure assignment

After the patient's case has been grouped into an MDC, the coder looks to see whether an operating room procedure was performed. Again, based on the documentation in the patient's record, the coder assigns ICD-9-CM codes to any and all procedures performed during the patient's stay.

Medical vs. surgical designation

Depending on the absence or presence of an operating room procedure, the coder then assigns the patient's case into either a medical or a surgical DRG.

Secondary diagnosis code assignment

A complication, or comorbidity (CC), is a secondary diagnosis that impacts DRG assignment. The presence of a CC implies that such a patient is more likely to consume more resources than a patient without a CC. Most DRGs are further divided into those with a complication or comorbidity. A CC is one way of further dividing the DRG; that is, for pneumonia there are two DRGs—simple pneumonia with CC and simple pneumonia without CC. The coder must carefully review all clinical documentation in the patient's record to identify any and all secondary diagnoses that are appropriately documented in the patient's record. The coder assigns an ICD-9-CM code to every secondary diagnosis.

It is appropriate to code a secondary diagnosis when:

- the condition is documented by the attending physician; and
- during the stay, the condition is either:
  - clinically evaluated
  - diagnostically tested
  - therapeutically treated
  - requires increasing nursing care or length of stay

Diagnosis-related group (DRG) assignment

Finally, after all codes have been assigned as described above, a DRG is assigned. Each DRG is assigned based on a relative weight (a number from approximately 0.4 to 3.5) that corresponds to the amount of resources the patients in that DRG, on average, consume during that hospital stay. The DRG then becomes a payment amount after the relative weight assigned to the DRG is multiplied by the hospital's "blended rate." The average blended rate for the nation is approximately $4,000. So for a DRG with a relative weight of 1.0, a hospital on average would be reimbursed $4,000. Appendix A lists all the current DRGs.

[1] Adapted from *Guidelines for Coding and Reporting,* CMS.

[2] Quote taken from the Uniform Hospital Discharge Data Set, maintained by the National Center for Health Statistics *(http://www.va.gov/publ/standard/healthfed/CDC_NCHS.html).*

CHAPTER 2

The Origins of Clinical Documentation in Patient Records

The Origins of Clinical Documentation in Patient Records

In 1964, Medicare was created as an entitlement system for U.S. citizens over age 65 and certain other classes of individuals. Shortly thereafter, the Medicare Conditions of Participation (COP) were created to determine the threshold criteria for hospitals qualified to receive Medicare and Medicaid payments. Many of the conditions focus on documentation requirements in the patient's record. These conditions have been updated and amended every year since 1964.

In addition to Medicare standards that govern the federal government's health insurance program, each state has adopted its own criteria for licensing hospitals within its borders to provide medical care. Every state licensure criteria list contains requirements for documentation. While state criteria can be more stringent than Medicare, none may be less stringent.

Finally, in the 1970s, accreditation by organizations such as the Joint Commission on Accreditation for Healthcare Organizations (JCAHO) began growing in popularity. The JCAHO has created its own set of criteria that a hospital must meet in order to obtain accreditation. Many of the JCAHO's criteria deal with documentation requirements in the patient's medical record. First, let's look at the COP, since they have pioneered documentation criteria in the inpatient medical record.

Medicare's Conditions of Participation

As previously stated, hospitals participating in Medicare must meet requirements outlined in the COP, which serve as the basis of survey activities for the federal government to determine whether a hospital qualifies for a provider agreement under Medicare and Medicaid. The COP are contained in Social Security and Medicare law in Title 42 of the *Code of Federal Regulations*.

Section 482.24 contains COP relating to medical record services in an acute care hospital. In particular, two standards in the medical record services section apply to documentation and related activities in the patient's medical record. While a lot of this information is primarily quantitative rather than qualitative, it is a jumping-off point for understanding documentation requirements. In many instances, the information provided in the COP can be used to infer qualitative content. The conditions that apply to inpatient documentation include standard B, standard C, delivery of service standard, and delivery of anesthesia services standard.

Standard B: Form and retention of the record

The hospital must maintain a medical record for each inpatient and outpatient service. Medical records must be accurately written, promptly completed, properly filed and retained, and accessible. The hospital must use a system of author identification and record maintenance that ensures the integrity of the authentication and protects the security of all record entries.

Standard C: Content of the record

The medical record must contain information to justify admission and continued hospitalization, support the diagnosis, and describe the patient's progress and response to medications and services. Included under this standard are the following clarifications:

1. All entries must be legible and complete, and must be authenticated and dated promptly by the person (identified by name and discipline) who is responsible for ordering, providing, or evaluating the service furnished.

   i. The author of each entry must be identified and must authenticate his or her entry.

   ii. Authentication may include signatures, written initials, or computer entry.

2. All records must document the following, as appropriate:

   i. Evidence of a physical examination, including a health history, performed no more than seven days prior to admission or within 48 hours after admission

   ii. Admitting diagnosis

iii. Results of all consultative evaluations of the patient and appropriate findings by clinical and other staff involved in the care of the patient

iv. Documentation of complications, hospital-acquired infections, and unfavorable reactions to drugs and anesthesia

v. Properly executed informed consent forms for procedures and treatments that are specified by the medical staff, or by federal or state law if applicable, to require written patient consent

vi. All practitioners' orders, nursing notes, reports of treatment, medication records, radiology, laboratory reports, vital signs, and other information necessary to monitor the patient's condition.

vii. Discharge summary with outcome of hospitalization, disposition of case, and provisions for follow-up care.

viii. Final diagnosis with completion of medical records within 30 days following discharge

Delivery of service standard

Surgical services must be consistent with needs and resources. Policies governing surgical care must be designed to assure the achievement and maintenance of high standards of medical practice and patient care.

1. There must be a complete history and physical work-up in the chart of every patient prior to surgery, except in emergencies. If this has been dictated, but not yet recorded in the patient's chart, there must be a statement to that effect and an admission note in the chart by the practitioner who admitted the patient.

2. A properly executed informed consent form for the operation must be in the patient's chart before surgery, except in emergencies.

3. The following equipment must be available to the operating room suites: call-in-system, cardiac monitor, resuscitator, defibrillator, aspirator, and tracheotomy set.

4. There must be adequate provisions for immediate postoperative care.

5. The operating room register must be complete and up to date.

6. An operative report describing techniques, findings, and tissues removed or altered must be written or dictated immediately following surgery and signed by the surgeon.

Delivery of anesthesia services standard

Anesthesia services must be consistent with needs and resources. Policies on anesthesia procedures must include the delineation of preanesthesia and postanesthesia responsibilities. The policies must ensure that the following are provided for each patient:

1. A preanesthesia evaluation by an individual qualified to administer anesthesia under paragraph (a) of this section, performed within 48 hours prior to surgery

2. An intraoperative anesthesia record

3. With respect to inpatients, a postanesthesia follow-up report that is written within 48 hours after surgery by the individual who administers the anesthesia

4. With respect to outpatients, a postanesthesia evaluation for proper anesthesia recovery performed in accordance with policies and procedures approved by the medical staff

Subsections of the COP

The COP also contain specific subsections relating to radiology, pharmacy, laboratory, and nuclear medicine. Each subsection addresses "acceptable standards of practice," and most contain specific provisions for "record keeping." For those subsections that do not contain information for record keeping, one must use the COP chapter on medical record services and documentation in general. The documentation guidelines in the medical record services section act as a "minimum documentation" requirement for the entire patient record. However, any subsection may require a greater degree of documentation as long as the requirements are spelled out within the specific subsection.

Emergency services

The only standard that applies to documentation in the emergency department subsection states, "There must be adequate medical and nursing personnel qualified in emergency care to meet the written emergency procedures and needs anticipated by the facility." The documentation referenced here is not specific clinical documentation, but rather documentation in the form of policies and procedures for emergency room care that every hospital must maintain. This condition focuses on the importance of internal policies and procedures, and lets providers know that they will be held to the standards that they create for themselves. It is important for all providers to keep in mind, as they create and validate policies and procedures, that if they create a standard for themselves that is higher than what the government requires, they will be held to that standard in the event of a review or audit.

Nuclear medicine

The nuclear medicine section contains a specific subsection that references "records." It states, "The hospital must maintain signed and dated reports of nuclear medicine interpretations, consultations, and procedures. The hospital must maintain copies of nuclear medicine reports for at least five years." These requirements focus more on quantity of documentation than quality, but nonetheless provide a source for documentation requirements that physicians may, at some point, question.

Radiologic services

The COP contain a subsection on radiologic services for records. It states, "The radiologist or other practitioner who performs radiology services must sign reports of his or her interpretations." Again, the information here is more quantitative than qualitative, but it still acts as a source for documentation requirements.

Pharmaceutical services

The pharmacy subsection states that "Drugs and biologicals not specifically prescribed as to time or number of doses must automatically be stopped after a reasonable time that is predetermined by the medical staff." This standard details that all orders for drugs must contain time and dose information. But it is important to note that the COP also contains a reference to the organization's internal policies and procedures. Specifically, the "medical staff" must determine what is a "reasonable time" to stop drugs that do not have the appropriate documentation contained in the order. In addition, the COP also contains a statement that "A formulary system must be established by the medical staff to assure quality pharmaceuticals at reasonable costs."

Laboratory services

The COP for laboratory services specifically state, "Emergency laboratory services must be available 24 hours a day. A written description of services provided must be available to the medical staff." The form and format of the listing of services have been a focus of compliance investigations in many hospitals. But as long as the list is complete and does not provide for the propensity to "unbundle" services, it will be in accordance with both the COP as well as compliance guidelines.

State licensure requirements

The following example of state documentation criteria comes from the regulations establishing the Arizona Board of Medical Education:

"Adequate records" means legible medical records containing, at a minimum, sufficient information to identify the patient, support the diagnosis, justify the treatment, accurately document the results, indicate advice and cautionary warnings provided to the patient and provide sufficient information for another practitioner to assume continuity of the patient's care at any point in the course of treatment.

Read more on this statute at *www.bomex.org/MDSTATUTES/title_32_update-new.htm#article2*. Read other states' requirements at *www.fsmb.org/members.htm*.

JCAHO

JCAHO refers to "completeness and timeliness" of information in its standards for hospitals.

Generally, JCAHO considers a patient's record to be complete when

- contents reflect the patients condition on arrival, diagnosis, test results, therapy, condition, in-hospital progress, and condition at discharge
- contents, including discharge summary, are assembled and authenticated
- all final diagnoses and complications are recorded without the use of symbols or abbreviations

Quality improvement organizations (QIOs [formerly "peer review organizations"]) also help define completeness of clinical documentation in the patient's record. For example, the PRO West, in one of its Payment Error Prevention Program studies, found the following:

- 31% of HIM departments surveyed reported that they generally have insufficient documentation to code the record accurately
- 10% of hospitals surveyed reported that they delayed coding records until the necessary documentation was available
- "There are instances when, due to time constraints, charts must be coded even while awaiting discharge summaries or responses to physician queries."

The *Official Guidelines for Coding and Reporting* (published by the Centers for Disease Control and Prevention) also address documentation quality and content. This resource states that "The importance of consistent and complete documentation in the medical record cannot be overemphasized. Without such documentation, the application of all coding guidelines is a difficult if not impossible task." (p. 7)

Finally, the issue of coding without a discharge summary plagues all HIM departments. It appears that, from an official resource perspective, there is no clear-cut guidance. This means that every HIM department must take it upon itself to ensure that it addresses the issue in the most effective manner through consistent coding policies and procedures. Here's what the official guidelines and other reliable resources have to say (or not say) about coding without a discharge summary on the record:

- Not addressed in Medicare COP
- Required for a "complete record" by JCAHO, but the coding issue is not addressed
- Acknowledged as "sometimes necessary" by some PROs for coding purposes
- Not specifically addressed by the OIG

Conclusion

In this chapter we have addressed the origins of clinical documentation—the COP—as well as the evolution of documentation standards. Many organizations are now involved in defining documentation standards. And even with all the attention and additional guideline development, HIM departments still have the same issues with physician documentation. Documentation is ambiguous, incomplete (especially when it comes to discharge summaries), and not as detailed as required for accurate coding. Although we need to be cognizant of the official guidelines and regulations for documentation, healthcare organizations will not find the answers to their clinical documentation woes in the words of the Office of the Inspector General (OIG) of the Department of Health and Human Services, Medicare COPs, or the JCAHO. However, by using this information as a springboard, each organization can begin to build the CDI program that will work for it. And within this book, we plan to share with you processes to design and implement CDI efficiently for your organization.

Figure 2.1 **Sources for Medical Record Content**

- **Medicare Conditions of Participation**
  http://www.access.gpo.gov/nara/cfr/waisidx_01/42cfr482_01.html
- **JCAHO**
  http://www.jcaho.org/search_frm.html
- **PRO Directory**
  http://www.hcfa.gov/quality/5b5.htm
- **Official Guidelines for Coding and Reporting (CDC)**
  http://www.cdc.gov/nchs/data/icdguide.pdf
- **OIG—3rd Party Billing Guidance (p. 7–fn. 48-51)**
  http://oig.hhs.gov/fraud/docs/complianceguidance/thirdparty.pdf

CHAPTER 3

The Physician and Medical Documentation

By John M. Williams, MD

The Physician and Medical Documentation

Written by John M. Williams, MD, an orthopedic surgeon with Bethlehem (PA) Orthopedic Associates.

"Documentation isn't so bad, except that it really cuts into your day." Most physicians have seen or heard this quote at one time or another during their professional lives. The quotation, usually accompanied by a cartoon character with either an enormous stack of paper or a roll of toilet paper, is meant to poke gentle fun at the time and energy spent completing medical documentation.

The majority of physicians have a love-hate relationship with most aspects of medical documentation: We love to hate it. We physicians are learning that like many other things that are not necessarily pleasant yet are beneficial to us (i.e., vaccinations, dieting, exercise, and giving up smoking), properly completed medical documentation is good for our patients, our hospitals, and ourselves.

In this chapter, I will discuss medical documentation from the physician's perspective, beginning with a review of physician training (both medical school and postgraduate training), an explanation of the relationship between the hospital and the physician, why documentation is important to physicians, and what motivates us to document the care of our patients.

Physician training

The future physician's training begins with a four-year college degree, culminating in either a bachelor of science or bachelor of arts degree. Required courses in biology, chemistry, organic chemistry, physics, and calculus are part of the premedical curriculum, but a science major is not required. The next step in the education of a physician is four years of medical school.

Chapter 3

The four-year medical school course is usually divided into two years of classroom study and two years of clinical study. Our primary goal as medical students is to learn all we can about the art and science of medicine in the allotted four years. Prompt and complete record keeping was stressed, including progress notes and history-and-physicals (H&Ps). I do not recall, however, any formal training concerning the medical business, which includes the subjects of coding, billing, and insurance. These were not discussed, and I am not sure we medical students would have retained any information on these topics if it had been presented. The relevance of this material became clear many years later, however.

Upon graduation, students are awarded the coveted "Doctorate of Medicine." However, for the graduates, the educational journey has just begun. All physicians who wish to practice clinical medicine or who wish to be licensed in medicine, must complete at least one year of postgraduate training. The goal of postgraduate medical education is to give the resident physician or fellow the maximum amount of practical information and experience in treating real patients. As in medical school, prompt, accurate, and complete medical record keeping is emphasized and expected. The resident physician is expected to dictate discharge summaries and operative summaries, in addition to completing H&Ps. There is little formal training in the preparation of these documents (other than the H&Ps); one "learns by doing." The resident physician views the medical record purely as a medical document, with little or no business or economic relevance. During my residency training, there was no formal training in the business or economics of medicine. Our department chairman was expected to make sure that his residents completed their charts in a timely manner. I remember one discussion in which the residents were complaining about having to complete their charts. His reply was "Complete your charts, or else. And no excuses or tricks. I tried all of them when I was a resident." Medical record documentation was a peripheral item in a full agenda of practical, patient-care–related teaching. The vast majority of my physician peers have experienced a similar lack of training in the business aspect of medicine during their years of medical school and residency training.

Like all good things, residency and fellowship training comes to an end. Most new physicians then enter clinical practice, the treating of patients. They are now referred to as "attending" physicians. The attending physician assumes full responsibility for, and ideally full control of, the care of his or her patients. In addition to the important clinical and medical aspects of patient care, the business and economic aspects now become relevant. This is true whether the attending physician is employed by a hospital or is in private practice. For most physicians, training in the business and economic aspects of medicine is received "on the job."

The relationship between an attending physician and the hospital where he or she is a member of the medical staff can be complex. This relationship can range from alliance to peaceful coexistence to confrontation. In almost all cases, the physician and the hospital need each other to survive, and although the relationship may not be a cordial one, it is a symbiotic one nonetheless. Physicians need the hospital to provide a place where they can refer patients for complex testing or procedures or where they can bring and care for patients who require inpatient care or surgery. It is essential for both physicians who are salaried employees of the hospital and for physicians who are self-employed, independent members of the medical staff.

The hospital, on the other hand, needs the revenues generated by the patients that physicians refer if it is to stay in operation. These revenues are used to purchase up-to-date equipment, to maintain the physical plant of the hospital, to hire and retain nursing and ancillary staff, and to pay for the other expenses of running the business of the hospital. Both for-profit and not-for-profit facilities need revenues to survive. It is mutually advantageous to both the physician and the hospital to ensure that the hospital receives the maximum allowable reimbursement for the services it provides. The medical record and the coding of the medical record play an important part in the reimbursement of both the hospital and the physician.

Documentation and the practice of medicine

Most physicians would rather spend their time in direct hands-on patient care than in medical record documentation. However, the importance of timely and complete medical records is becoming more apparent to most physicians. This documentation process is motivated by and mediated through government agencies, insurance companies, managed care companies, and hospital administrations. These organizations motivate physicians predominantly through fear. Fear of not being paid and fear of being excluded from Medicare or another payer's program are probably the two biggest motivators for physicians to act and to cooperate. The mediation of the process comes in various forms, including the hospital management team and the utilization review (UR) staff from the insurance companies and managed care companies. The primary job of these UR individuals is to identify when "protocol" has not been met, which could result in a potentially noncovered episode of care. Such a finding, of course, is a win for the managed care organization and a loss for the physician.

In all fairness, many managed care companies do focus on what is in the "best interest of the patient." As a result, these companies will attempt to work cooperatively with the physicians to ask for additional documentation or information to support a patient's hospital stay, surgery, or other episode of care.

Timely and complete documentation is important for several reasons. These include continuity of patient care, organizational/business needs, and medical-legal issues.

Continuity of patient care

From the physician's point of view, continuity of patient care is the most important reason for timely and complete medical documentation. Continuity of care means that all members of the patient-care team know the relevant information about a patient and the pertinent details of what the other members of the team are trying to accomplish. The permanent record of the patient's care, which is documented in each patient's chart or medical record, is the primary source of and repository for that information. Relevant information and pertinent details regarding the patient are shared by the patient's attending physician (the primary physician), consulting physicians (who advise on other medical/surgical issues), nurses, therapists, and case managers/social workers. Important information is shared among similar practitioners as well (i.e., physician-to-physician) and different practitioners (i.e., nurse-to-physician). The goal is that all practitioners understand each other and that they serve the patient's best interests.

Organizational/business needs

Proper medical record documentation also serves the organizational needs of the hospital and the physician. The first of these organizational needs are financial in nature, because without the revenues generated by patient services, the hospital could not exist and the physician could not operate. The governmental agencies, insurance companies, and managed care organizations who pay for the vast majority of healthcare in this country require proof that services actually were rendered before paying for them. This proof resides in the patient's medical record. "If it isn't documented, it didn't happen," is the mantra of today's healthcare payers. Lack of timely and complete medical record documentation can and does cost hospitals and physicians millions of dollars in lost revenue for care that they provided but for which they were not reimbursed.

Another organizational need that medical record documentation impacts is planning, both short- and long-term. Hospital administrators and their staffs study the information in medical records to help them plan for the future. Their planning may address immediate, short-term issues such as staffing levels (particularly nursing), supplies, and equipment. Or it may attempt to answer long-range questions such as "Should we build a new hospital wing?" or "buy another MRI machine?" or "invest in new services or programs?" Incomplete or nonexistent documentation may mean that planners do not have accurate information on which to base their plans.

Certification and licensure are other organizational activities in which medical record documentation plays an important part, because all hospitals and outpatient facilities require a state license to operate. These licenses must be renewed regularly, a process that may include inspections, either announced or unannounced. Poor medical record documentation is a guaranteed way to fail an inspection, which can result in major licensing problems for the organization and major headaches for the administrators of that organization. In addition to being licensed, almost all hospitals and most major outpatient facilities are certified by the JCAHO. This certification is a benchmark of quality, and it is required by most healthcare payers before they will reimburse a hospital or outpatient facility for services rendered. The JCAHO conducts an exhaustive inspection of the facility in question prior to certifying or recertifying that facility. As with licensure, timely and complete medical record documentation is required for certification by the JCAHO, and poor documentation can be a cause for withholding or limiting certification.

Medical and legal issues

Proper medical record documentation is also important in the medical and legal venue because it plays a key role in medical malpractice litigation. Lack of timely or complete medical record documentation is a serious problem for the medical/legal defense team. As with billing and reimbursement, "if it isn't documented, it didn't happen." This motto applies particularly to the issue of informed consent. Medical record documentation should contain the thought processes and treatment rationale of the treating physician(s), which can be very useful to the medical defense team in litigation.

Medical documentation, the physician, and competing priorities

In spite of tremendous scientific advances, man has not discovered a way to pack more than 24 hours in a day. Most physicians—and most people in any occupation—have more things to do in any given day than there is time to do them. As physicians, most of our professional time is spent caring for patients in the hospital, in the operating room, or in the office. We spend increasing amounts of time engaged in the business of medicine, which includes the business of running a practice, as well as serving on hospital committees. In an era of declining reimbursements and rising costs, physicians and hospitals must pay more attention to the business details of medicine in order to continue to practice the patient care of medicine.

Most physicians would put increased personal time and time with their families at the top of the list of things they desire. This is especially true for young physicians just out of residency training and physicians in the middle or nearing the end of their careers. Much further down the list is the wish for "more time to spend on medical record completion." In spite of this lack of enthusiasm, hospital administrators and the physicians who participate in hospital administration have tried, and continue to try, to motivate their medical staff colleagues to achieve timely and accurate medical record completion. In the past, this has been on a voluntary basis, with gentle reminders to "please complete your charts." If a JCAHO inspection were imminent, the reminder might be more urgent, but cooperation on the part of the physician was still voluntary.

Enter the new millennium. Timely and accurate medical record completion now is a necessity, not an option. Truth is, it always was a necessity, but hospitals, and particularly physicians, did not assign a high priority to medical documentation. Hospitals now must maintain a high percentage of medical records completed on time—or else. "Or else" can include inadequate reimbursement for services rendered, Medicare audits and fines, loss or modification of its operating license, or poor performance and loss of certification on a JCAHO inspection. Hospital administrators have gotten the message and have passed it on to the physicians on their hospital's medical staff.

How has that message been delivered? Most hospitals have begun enforcing sections in their bylaws that have been in effect for many years mandating suspension of medical staff privileges for physicians who do not complete their medical records in a timely fashion. Suspension of privileges means no patients admitted and no surgeries performed. At some hospitals, this suspension includes all physicians of a group if one physician is delinquent, which can bring a medical practice to a grinding halt in a hurry. This draconian measure effectively serves to get the attention of the offending physician and produces the desired result—prompt medical record completion.

In years past, when suspension for incomplete medical records was not enforced, the suspension list at one of our local hospitals might include 30 names and at least several members of each of the larger group practices. Because administrators have begun to enforce bylaws regarding incomplete medical records through suspending privileges, the list now includes five or fewer names, and it rarely includes physicians who do a major portion of their work at that hospital. Thus, the hospital administration has successfully advanced the position of medical record completion on the physician's list of competing priorities.

Conclusion

Medical record keeping is here to stay. Even with the advent of electronic medical records, physicians must still prepare (dictate or write) and sign the pertinent documents. Some (mostly older) physicians are still not convinced that the electronic medical record is a step forward. Whether paper or electronic, however, the medical record must be completed. We physicians cannot go back to the "good old days" of incomplete, delinquent medical records. Our hospital administrators will not allow it, and it is in our best interests not to go backwards.

CHAPTER 4

Assessing Documentation in Your Organization

Assessing Documentation in Your Organization

The documentation audit

Before embarking on a full-fledged documentation improvement program, you need to review your documentation habits to spot weaknesses. This review, the documentation audit, will give you your "baseline" findings, from which all of your initial planning will emanate. All your subsequent actions depend on this review, so it's imperative that you document it thoroughly and conduct it with a high degree of precision.

> In the documentation audit, you determine whether the physician's documentation in the patient's record provides the highest possible degree of specificity and clarity to ensure the most accurate diagnostic coding.

The documentation audit is not a coding audit. Rather, it addresses documentation problems affecting coding that a retrospective physician query cannot cure. In the audit, you identify these problems, which include documentation that is incomplete, unclear, nonspecific, and focused on the symptoms rather than on the etiology of disease. The audit identifies documentation in the patient's record that, if clarified or further specified by the attending physician, could have an impact on the ICD-9-CM diagnostic codes assigned to the patient and, in turn, on the DRG assignment and payment to the hospital for the patient's stay.

Retrospective versus concurrent documentation review

The first decision that you need to make is whether you will conduct the review concurrently or retrospectively. A concurrent, or prospective, review means that the auditors review and comment on the documentation in the patient's record while the patient is still on the nursing unit. A retrospective review means that the auditors review the documentation after the patient has been discharged. Although it is possible to conduct the documentation review on either a concurrent or retrospective basis, the benefits of the concurrent documentation review far outweigh the administrative efficiencies of the retrospective review.

Retrospective reviews

There are pros and cons to conducting the documentation review in either a retrospective or a concurrent manner. First, let's examine the retrospective review. It is easier to conduct from an administrative perspective. Records of discharged patients are readily available, and the reviewer does not have to take up healthcare providers' time. During a retrospective review, auditors have enough room to perform the review on the nursing unit. In addition, the sample selection can be performed using statistically valid sampling techniques, including stratification. For example, every provider can be proportionately represented within the review. Thus, the results of the review can be extrapolated over the entire population of patients and physicians more easily than the results of a concurrent review.

The retrospective review process limits the provider's ability to amend the documentation under review, however. In fact, in many cases it is too late to correct documentation errors once reviewers have identified them. Documentation issues can simply be denoted as gaps that, had the physician documented in greater detail, might have resulted in a change in code assignment.

The fact that the reviewer is working with many unknowns in this process means that the results of the review need to be tempered to offset these unknowns. When a reviewer tempers results for unknown factors, he or she applies clinical expertise to the situation in the case of missing documentation. Because the clinician was not actually present during the provision of care but rather is only reading the record, the clinician needs to temper the information that may be missing in the patient's record with his or her expert clinical knowledge and, in some cases, clinical intuition.

For example, let's say that, during a documentation audit, a reviewer audits the records of ten simple pneumonia cases. Two of those cases make vague references to facts about a patient's case. One refers to a patient's transfer from a skilled nursing facility, and another refers to an immunocompromised condition that might lead a clinician to suspect that the patient's pneumonia was caused by either a bacterial agent or the aspiration of foreign material.

These two cases lacked enough documentation to support a retrospective query. In a concurrent audit, a clinician might have spotted this gap in documentation, consulted the physician, and corrected it during the patient's stay. You can't improve documentation in cases like this, but you can quantify roughly how much documentation improvement a physician ought to make. In this case, 20% of the cases appeared to support some improved documentation.

You can temper your results so as not to overstate them: multiply the percentage of cases that need better documentation by 50% (or less if you feel more comfortable). You may want to temper the above finding by 25%. This means that the documentation in approximately 5% (20% x 25%) of all of the simple pneumonia cases could use improvement. The process of tempering findings, though not an exact science by any means, can validate retrospective documentation audit findings.

Concurrent reviews

Let's turn now to the pros and cons of a concurrent review. Unlike a retrospective review, a concurrent review can lead to actual changes in documentation. As a result, the findings of a concurrent review may be more reliable, in some ways, than those of the retrospective review.

The concurrent audit is performed on the nursing unit while the patient is still in house. It involves reviewing physician documentation almost immediately after the physician provides the documentation. Ideally, in a concurrent documentation review, the reviewer can request more details from the attending physician in cases where the clinical documentation needs improvement. Then, the reviewer should follow up to ensure that the physician has complied. If the physician adds documentation that impacts coding and DRG assignment, these numbers become part of the significant findings.

The prospective review has several weaknesses, however. First, clinicians cannot control the sample type. The concurrent review examines only the records of inpatients that happen to be on the nursing units at the time when the review is conducted. In addition, the findings may be tainted by what has come to be known in social research as the "Hawthorne Factor," a concept that arose during social experiments in the late 1930s. It determines, among other things, that the results of a study can be greatly affected if the subjects under study know that they are being observed. Physicians who know that they are being audited may document better than they normally would, thereby skewing the results.

Finally, as with the retrospective review results, even concurrent review results must be tempered. Clinicians on the units or auditors may identify some potential for documentation improvement when they look at a patient record, but there is no way to know whether the physician would have made any improvements without the intervention of the clinician. You need to account for this in your study results. To determine what the likely documentation results would have been without the audit, compare the projected results against actual results. In general, you can assume that approximately 30% of the documentation improvement that resulted from review findings would have occurred anyway. Therefore, temper your findings by about 30%.

For example, during a retrospective review, the reviewer asks surgeons whether ten surgical cases had secondary complications and comorbidities. In 30% of the cases, the physicians said yes. By tempering the results, one might assume that approximately 10% of all surgical cases are under-documented underdocumented for complications or comorbidities that would impact coding, DRG assignment, and reimbursement.

Both the retrospective and concurrent documentation audit processes have their strengths and weaknesses. In general, if you can perform the review concurrently, the results will be more reliable. Whichever method you choose, temper your results. This way, you avoid setting unrealistically high targets for documentation improvement.

Sample selection

As with any review, you will need to select a representative sampling. Ask yourself the following questions when you select your sample:

1. What payors should we include in the review?
2. What providers should we include in the review?
3. Do we want to focus on certain documentation issues up front, or should we include all documentation concerns in the initial review?

While every organization must respond to these questions according to its own organizational philosophy, we recommend that, initially, the review focus only on payors that reimburse inpatients according to the PPS. By including non-PPS payors, you may overstate your projections for the benefits of a documentation improvement program. In addition, we recommend that all providers and all documentation concerns be addressed from the beginning. Except in large university-teaching institutions, splitting off different documentation issues and providers will inevitably result in a less focused, underwhelming documentation improvement effort.

Retrospective sample selection

Retrospective sample selection should involve a simple random sample for all inpatient cases with a potential for documentation improvement. Cases with the potential for documentation improvement can easily be identified based upon by the coding and DRG assignment for the patient cases upon discharge.

Certain codes are considered to be potentially "nonacute" principal diagnoses. For example, a patient is admitted with a condition that resembles epistaxis. If that condition is coded, the analyst will reach one of the following conclusions: This patient should not have been admitted to this facility, since people aren't admitted to acute care for nosebleeds. More likely, however, the physician did not adequately document the etiology of the epistaxis, which could have been hypertension or a bleeding disorder.

If documented appropriately, this patient's case would not have had a principal diagnosis of epistaxis, but rather hypertension or coagulopathy, depending on the situation.

This method of sample selection will ensure that you have a good number of cases to review in all clinical areas and from all providers. To determine the number of cases that you to include in your sample, we recommend that you refer to Dr. Wang's sample selection table, which is shown in Figure 4.1. This table is an easy-to-use guide to ensure that you have the correct number of cases in your sample selection to guarantee a representative and statistically sound sample.

Concurrent sample selection

Concurrent sample selection is slightly more challenging than retrospective sample selection. First, you need to define the time period for your review and stick to it. For example, if you determine ahead of time that the review will be performed from January 10th through 14th, you need to keep to the parameters that you have defined. Then, you need to determine the number of cases that should be reviewed. You can use the sample selection table previously provided in Figure 4.1 as a guide. But, keep in mind that in a concurrent review, your sample is a convenience sample, not a random one, so the numbers in the sample selection table will not guarantee any degree of statistical significance. You may want to set parameters for review in nursing units

Figure 4.1

Desired Sample Size for a Simple Random-Sample Survey from a Given Population and Permissible Error at the 95% Confidence Level

Population	Sample Size and Permissible Error				
	±.05	±.04	±03	±.02	±.01
100	73	81	88	94	99
200	115	136	158	179	194
300	143	176	215	255	287
400	162	206	261	324	378
500	176	229	301	386	466
600	187	248	334	443	551
700	195	264	363	495	634
800	202	277	388	543	715
900	208	288	410	588	794
1,000	213	297	429	629	871
2,000	238	349	547	917	1,544
3,000	248	371	601	1,082	2,079
4,000	254	382	633	1,189	2,514
5,000	257	390	654	1,264	2,875
6,000	259	395	668	1,320	3,180
7,000	261	399	679	1,362	3,440
8,000	262	402	687	1,396	3,666
9,000	263	404	694	1,424	3,862
10,000	263	406	699	1,447	4,035
20,000	267	414	724	1,559	5,055
30,000	268	417	733	1,601	5,520
40,000	269	418	738	1,623	5,787
50,000	269	419	741	1,636	5,959

Source: Wang, MQ, Fitzhugh, E & Westerfield, RC (1995) "Determining Sample Sizes for Simple Random Surveys" 19(3): 53 – 56. *Health Values*

where the patients are housed during their stay. For example, using a parameter such as sampling every PPS patient in an odd-numbered bed helps make the convenience sample more random. In general, you should include at least the number of cases recommended by the sample selection table, if not more.

Record review

Although the individual performing the documentation audit must have significant experience with the PPS system and the types of diagnoses and procedures that impact DRG assignment, record review for a documentation improvement audit is different from record review for a coding audit. The primary goal of a documentation audit is to improve documentation. Generally, the improvement falls into one of the following categories:

1. Principal diagnosis:

    - needs more detail
    - needs documentation for etiology (in the case of a symptom documented as the principal diagnosis)
    - creates a conflict or needs clarification (in the case of a conflict between the attending physician and a consulting physician)

2. Secondary diagnosis:

    - supporting clinical documentation—needs physician documentation
    - supporting nursing documentation—needs physician documentation
    - supporting physician documentation—needs clarification

3. Procedure:

    - additional detail needed

Therefore, the review will focus on these types of documentation issues. Any time you identify a documentation issue, record it on the audit form. A type of audit form called a Query Tracking Sheet can be found in Figure 4.2. In the case of a concurrent review audit, record whether the physician makes changes to the documentation as a result of a concurrent query. In each case, the audit form should also collect the original DRG assignment (assuming no documentation improvement had occurred) and

Figure 4.2

Query Tracking Sheet

Date of Admission			
Review Date			
Patient Account #			
Patient Name			
Unit			
Principal Diagnosis			
Principal Procedure			
Working DRG			
Relative Weight			
Pre—Query Payment			
Type of Query			
Query Results			
Discharge DRG			
Relative Weight			
Post—Query Payment			
Payment Difference (Pre—Post)			

the changed DRG assignment, assuming that the requested documentation improvement has occurred. The review for each record in the documentation improvement audit should determine if there is any room for improvement. If there is, the review should determine how that improvement would benefit the hospital.

Data collection

The reviewer must collect data once the record review is completed. Data collection can be performed manually or with the use of an automated system like Microsoft Excel© or Access. Ultimately, you need to collect the data to show how your suggested changes would affect coding, DRG assignment, and the case-mix index of the hospital. The number of changes and types of changes should be collected. Also, which DRGs—or ideally, which medical and surgical specialties—are most likely impacted by the improved documentation should be gleaned from the review data. See Figure 4.3 for a sample aggregate data collection form. Remember to temper all of your aggregate analysis results by decreasing impact somewhere between 30% and 50% of

Figure 4.3 **CDI Opportunities by Specialty**

Specialty	# of cases w/potential	Expected change rate	Expected CMI impact
General Medicine	884	30%	.0085
Cardiology	558	33%	.0062
General Surgery	242	47%	.0049
Orthopedic Surgery	318	32%	.0041
Gynecology	346	31%	.0037
Neurology	278	28%	.0019
Urology	83	26%	.0008
Totals	2,709		.0301

[1] numbers based on Sample Hospital Medicare Inpatient data 07/01/01 through 12/31/01

Figure 4.3

CDI Assessment Data Results[1] (continued)

Medical Cases with potential for documentation improvement

Diagnosis/Procedure/DRG Title	Annual Discharges[2]
TIA	120
Dizziness	22
Bronchitis & asthma	60
AMI without major complication	100
Syncope	80
Chest pain	190
Back pain	70
Medical DRGs without complications/comorbidities (various DRGs)	1,0781[1]
Total medicine cases with potential for documentation improvement	1,720

[1]Data results are based on a review of aggregate Medicare data provided by sample

[2]based on sample hospital inpatient data 7/01/01 – 12/31/01

[3]includes DVT, arrhythmia, syncope, GI bleed, uncomplicated ulcer, bowel obstruction, cellulitis, dehydration

UTI as principal diagnosis all without a complicating/cormorbid condition

Surgical Cases with potential for documentation improvement

Diagnosis/Procedure/DRG Title	Annual Discharges[2]
AAA repair/other major vascular procedures	22
Minor vascular surgery	63
Intestinal surgery	52
Stomach surgery	16
Gallbladder surgery	24
Hip fracture repair	53
Back surgery	190
Other orthopedic surgery	73
Minor orthopedic surgery	17
Mastectomy	26
Minor lung procedures	20

Figure 4.3 **CDI Assessment Data Results[1] (continued)**

Surgical cases with potential for documentation improvement

Diagnosis/Procedure/DRG Title	Annual Discharges[2]
Male transurethral procedures	133
Hysterectomies	300
Total Surgical cases	989
Total cases with potential for documentation improvement	2,709

[1] Data results are based on a review of aggregate Medicare data provided by sample hospital
[2] based on sample hospital inpatient data 07/01/01 – 12/31/01

Top 15 Medicare attending physicians

Physician ID	# of Medicare Admissions	% of Total Medicare Admissions
30155	155	2.34%
00972	153	2.31%
00835	152	2.30%
00699	101	1.53%
00204	91	1.37%
11580	83	1.25%
11263	81	1.22%
00088	77	1.16%
11250	71	1.07%
00200	66	1.00%
00455	65	0.98%
13581	64	0.97%
31849	56	0.85%
11443	52	0.79%
94750	51	0.77%
Totals	1,318	19.91%

Figure 4.3

CDI Assessment Data Results[1](continued)

Attending Physicians with Greatest Potential for Documentation Improvement

Physician ID	# Cases with DI Potential	CMI Impact
30155	48	.0010
00204	25	.0005
00699	24	.0005
11580	24	.0005
11263	21	.0004
00088	20	.0004
94750	20	.0004
00200	19	.0004
13581	19	.0004
54759	18	.0004
00479	17	.0003
11132	17	.0003
11250	17	.0003
11569	17	.0011
24530	16	.0003
Totals	**322**	**.0072**

Top 15 Medicare Attending Physicians also on DI List = ✗

Physician ID	# of Medicare Admissions	% of Total Medicare Admissions	On both lists 66%
30155	155	2.34%	✗
00972	153	2.31%	
00835	152	2.30%	
00699	101	1.53%	✗
00204	91	1.37%	✗
11580	83	1.25%	✗
11263	81	1.22%	✗
00088	77	1.16%	✗
11250	71	1.07%	✗
00200	66	1.00%	✗
00455	65	0.98%	
13581	64	0.97%	✗
31849	56	0.85%	
11443	52	0.79%	
94750	51	0.77%	✗
Totals	**1,318**	**19.91%**	**10/66%**

actual findings, so as not to overstate the expected results of a documentation improvement program. (Tempering is discussed in detail in the previous section on "retrospective vs. concurrent review.")

Data analysis

Once you have collected the data from the review, study them closely to determine what the results of the review may indicate. Hopefully, you will have collected data that shows that there will be some impact to coding, DRG assignment, and reimbursement to the hospital. The degree of impact should drive your decision regarding the implementation of a documentation improvement program. In addition to identifying the proposed impact that a documentation improvement program will have on DRG assignment, you should seek to analyze the data at lower levels as well. For example, what does the data tell you about specific medical or surgical specialties? If, for example, you found that 30% of the DRGs with real potential for documentation improvement were in the cardiovascular medical DRGs, then you should mention in your analysis that cardiologists, as specialists, could contribute significantly to improving documentation in the hospital.

Report preparation

Your report preparation should include an initial executive summary like the one in Figure 4.4. This executive summary should show the projected impact that a documentation improvement program would have on your organization. The extent of the impact, of course, is based on the findings of the documentation audit. Then, you should present data in a format that includes a lot of specificity from the audit review. This detailed review presentation gives credibility to your projections. There are various ways that you can present the data, but you may want to consider providing the following tables, which point out opportunities for documentation improvement by:

- Diagnosis
- Procedure
- Medical and surgical specialties
- Physician

Finally, include recommendations accompanied by a cost-benefit analysis to support your recommendations. For example, if you calculated that an effective documentation improvement program would provide an additional $500,000 in gross revenue to your facility, follow up by showing how to implement that program. Your program

Figure 4.4 **Projected Results of an Implemented CDI Program**

Executive Summary

Annual Medicare discharges	12,000
Medicare case mix index (CMI):	1.5200[1]
Projected Impact of documentation improvement initiative on annual CMI:	+.0301[2]
Dollar value for each 1% of CMI:	XXX[3]
Projected impact of documentation improvement on annual revenue:	XXX[3]

[1]Medicare case mix index information obtained from the American Hospital Directory
[2]Applying a 90% confidence interval, CMI change range = .0273 - .0333
[3]Information unavailable at the time of analysis

Note: All information based on data provided by sample hospital for discharges 7/1/01 through 12/31/01

CDI Improvement Assessment

Record Review Results

Time period reviewed	07/01/01 – 12/31/01[1]	
Number of Medicare cases in time period	11,675	
Medical	7,369	63%
Surgical	4,254	37%
Number of cases with opportunity for documentation improvement	2,709	
Medical	1,720	64%
Surgical	989	36%
Total annual CMI Impact[1]	.0301	
Total approximate annual financial impact for cases reviewed	XXX[2]	

[1]Data was extrapolated from time period provided for a 12-month period
[2]Information unavailable at the time of analysis

Figure 4.4 **Projected Results of an Implemented CDI Program (cont.)**

CDI Assessment

Data measure	Data Results[1] Current	Projected
Total Medicare CMI:	1.520	1.550
CMI for medical cases:	1.041	1.058
CMI for surgical cases:	2.562	2.575
Surgical CMI as driver of overall CMI:	246%	243%

should include projected costs, which, of course, should be less than the additional revenue to your facility.

Analysis of documentation in your organization

Beyond the analysis in the documentation improvement audit report, you should provide additional analysis to your administration to support the documentation improvement program. In particular, this type of additional analysis can support a specific focus. One of the most helpful analyses that you can perform involves a review of the highest admitting physicians in your facility. Next, you can perform an analysis of the physicians who appear to have the greatest need for documentation improvement. You can then combine these two reports to show which physicians are both high admitters and poor documenters. This type of analysis can show the administration, in many cases, that an initial focus on educating certain physicians can result in a high return on investment to the organization. We address the specifics of such education in Chapter 5.

In this analysis, it helps to refer to our documentation model, referenced on page 12 in Chapter 1. The model incorporates all of the people involved in the documentation process. We address their roles, or potential roles, in improving documentation in the following section.

Go to the source

In addition to analyzing records, you should go to the source—the physicians—in the assessment phase of your documentation improvement program. The health information management (HIM) director and other members of the HIM department are some of the professionals who are most familiar with the documentation habits of physicians. Certainly, the HIM professional knows which physicians are, at least subjectively, considered "good documenters," as well as those who are likely to cooperate when asked to provide additional documentation on an inpatient record. The process that we call "rating your physicians" is one of the pre-clinical documentation improvement (CDI) program activities in which you should engage.

Depending on the size of your organization, you should be able to identify the top 100 to 250 attending physicians for inpatient cases. You may want to further refine your numbers based upon the top admitters for PPS-based patients, just to determine if there are any significant differences between the two lists. After you have identified these physicians, you will want to begin the rating process. The categories into which you will place each physician are (1) leaders/early adopters, (2) late adopters, and (3) nonadopters.

Leaders/early adopters

Every hospital has physician leaders who not only do what they are asked to do, but are willing to help when asked. They are the physicians who serve on committees and always show up for meetings. Granted, these physicians may be few in number, but it is necessary to identify them because they will serve an integral role in the CDI process. Physician leaders can be planted in meetings and presentations to show support for the program when it's needed the most. These physicians can be used to present portions of educational sessions when credibility is at stake or the hospital is faced with adversity from nonadopters.

Late adopters

Late adopters are physicians who may be skeptical of new programs and projects but who in time have usually bought into the programs that truly have an impact on the organization. The support of these physicians is key and can actually have a larger impact than that of the physician leaders, especially in trying to win over the nonadopters. For example, when a nonadopter physician is present at an educational session that is run by or supported by a physician leader, the nonadopter is likely to think to himself or herself, "Dr. Smith is one of the administration's puppets." Hence, Dr. Smith's presence may have little impact on the nonadopter's attitude. However, if Dr. Jones, who is also a late adopter, is leading the meeting, the nonadopter may take more notice of this and think, "Gee, Dr. Jones doesn't usually show such support for these types of programs. Maybe they're onto something here."

Nonadopters

Your nonadopters will most likely be divided into two groups: those who will eventually buy into some level of the program and those who never will. You will also need to identify those nonadopters who are also high admitters. If you have nonadopters who are also high admitters, you will want to initiate one-on-one sessions or other workable solutions in order to glean results from the activities of these essential but nonsupportive physicians. Nonadopters who are also low admitters are probably not worth any additional effort. It is important to keep reassessing high admitters on an ongoing basis. You do not want one of your nonadopter low admitters to suddenly have a large number of patient admissions without your being aware of it so you can take appropriate measures.

The attending physician

Your CDI program should also address how your organization views the duties of the attending physician. This is an important concept because in many organizations there is, even today, some confusion about the documentation responsibilities of the attending physician. Furthermore, some organizations have not settled on a policy at all. The issue as to whether the attending physician is ultimately responsible for all documentation in an inpatient record first came to a head in 1994. That year, the government eliminated, through the Paperwork Reduction Act, the requirement that the attending physician had to attest to all of the coding and documentation in the patient's record—the basis for the Medicare bill—by affixing his or her signature to that record. The problem with this administrative change was that the elimination of the signature requirements was the only change that was made. In essence, the new law did not excuse the attending physician from having to attest to the documentation and coding in the patient's record; that was, and still is, required. As a practical matter, we can only code only from documentation that is either provided or agreed to by the attending physician.

Further support for the attending physician's responsibility for documentation can be found in the *Official Guidelines for Coding and Reporting*. The guidelines explicitly state that, in the case of a conflict in a patient's record between the documentation of the attending physician and that of any other physician treating the patient (i.e., consultant, pathologist, etc.), the attending physician's notations always takes take precedence. To take this one step further, consider the attending internal medicine physician who orders a consult from a neurologist for a patient with "dizzy spells." The consultant documents that the patient has an impending cerebrovascular accident (CVA), but the attending physician fails to corroborate the diagnosis. In this case, the neurologist's documentation, even though more definitive (and probably correct, because she or he is the expert), cannot be coded. Why? Because the attending physicians did not state "CVA," or document something like "Agree with neuro consult."

To assess the obstacles to documentation improvement, analyze your organization's policies regarding the attending physician's documentation. We have provided our interpretation of the official guidance and legislation above. But in any event, you need to make certain that your organization is comfortable with its current process regarding attending physician documentation requirements before going forward with a CDI program. If you are not comfortable with your policy, you will need to revise and implement it prior to proceeding.

Other physicians who treat the patient

Regardless of your organization's policy on the attending physician's documentation, you will still need to assess the other physicians who may treat or diagnose the patient. Whether you rely on their documentation or not, the presence of rich, detailed documentation from these individuals can mean the difference between documentation improvement and no change at all. Make a list of these physicians and rate them as well. Some of the categories of physicians who will fall into this group include:

- Radiologists/nuclear medicine physicians
- Pathologists
- Infectious disease physicians
- Diagnostic cardiologists
- Emergency department physicians
- Anesthesiologists

Depending on the organization, many additional physicians may fall into this group. If they are employed by the hospital, you will more easily enlist their cooperation than with outside physicians. Nonetheless, it will be necessary to divide these physicians into leaders/early adopters, late adopters, and nonadopters to determine how to approach them for their participation in the program.

Hospitalists

The "hospitalists" that we refer to in this book are physicians who are employed by acute care hospitals for the sole purpose of providing care to inpatients. In hospitalist programs, a hospital will hire physicians and then offer, as a service to the physicians in the community, the hospitalists' services to care for those physicians' patients when they need to be admitted as inpatients. The programs are not mandatory and are generally seen as a good public relations tool for hospitals that implement them. Internal medicine physicians who have busy practices mostly use them. For the community physician, the hospitalist program allows internal medicine physicians to concentrate on their office practice. For the hospital, the hospitalist program allows greater control over issues like length of stay and documentation. Therefore, in assessing your organization's potential for a successful documentation improvement program, you will want to include the role of hospitalists, if you have them.

Identify clinical supporters

Who will be the clinical supporters for your CDI program besides physicians? We can safely assume that if the CDI program is left in the hands of physicians, it will not succeed. It is the hospital's responsibility to provide support, in the form of other clinical personnel, for the CDI program. Therefore. in assessing your organization's preparedness and likelihood to succeed with CDI, you will need to honestly determine if you have the nonphysician clinical support in place to proceed If not, you will need to determine how you can create this support.

The implementation of a CDI program will not be exactly the same in any two hospitals. Therefore, the clinical supporters who provide the foundation for CDI in one hospital may differ from the clinical supporters in another hospital. Some of the clinical supporters who can play a role in documentation improvement include the following:

- Case managers
- Nurse unit managers

- UR/discharge planning staff
- Quality Assurance/Quality Improvement staff
- Clinical outcomes managers

Identify nonclinical supporters

To succeed, the CDI program must also have support from more than the clinical arena. Clearly, as we stated before, CDI is an organization-wide activity. It touches literally every piece of the organization in some way. There are many nonclinical experts who play essential roles in the ongoing CDI process. These professionals support the clinical piece by providing data to support and track the clinical process and expertise in interpreting the impact and effect of the CDI process. Some of the individuals who need to be included in your assessment, in terms of resources and assistance, are

- Credentialed HIM coding professionals
- Case mix managers
- Information system specialists
- Financial/reimbursement professionals
- Financial/reimbursement professionals

The final assessment

The final assessment should include a review of all of the elements we have addressed in this chapter. You should rate your organization on a scale of 1 to 5 in each of the aforementioned areas. Perform this final assessment by using the CDI preparedness assessment form, shown in Figure 4.4. We have quantified scores that indicate your organization is prepared to proceed with documentation improvement. In cases where you are not yet prepared, the assessment form will indicate where you need to provide additional resources or policy issues that need to be resolved before you should proceed.

CHAPTER 5

The Role of Education in Documentation Improvement

The Role of Education in Documentation Improvement

Chapter 5

In any new program or process, education plays a central role. This applies to the implementation of a clinical documentation improvement program as well. But, because the issues that impact CDI are constantly in flux, education is a continuous part of CDI programming. Therefore, when assessing the educational portion of your CDI program, you should do so in two phases: First, assess the initial education needs of your CDI team and population; then plan how to manage the ongoing process. You will need to answer the following questions for both the initial training as well as the ongoing CDI education:

- Whom to educate?
- What subjects should the education program should include?
- How to educate?
- When to educate?

Whom to educate?

You will need to educate everyone involved in the CDI program, including all of the individuals addressed in the previous chapter. You can roll out your training in the most efficient manner by dividing groups of individuals who need training into similar groups by job type or by clinical specialty. You can also divide training sessions into "most general" and "most specialized."

General introductory session

Most individuals involved in any way in documentation improvement need to know certain general information. This material could be covered in a mandatory two-hour session for all nonphysician CDI participants, and perhaps in a 30-minute session for all physicians.

Employed physicians

In general, employed physicians should be educated before community-based physicians, partly because you will get more cooperation from the former group. By "employed physicians," we mean every physician group that may be employed by the organization. The faster you can provide these physicians with the resources to begin making a difference in documentation, the sooner your organization will begin to see a return on investment. In addition, these physicians can influence their nonemployed peers. In many organizations, employed physicians can have a broad reach. This group can include the following practitioners:

- Primary care physicians
- Other hospital-owned physician groups
- Emergency department physicians
- Radiologists
- Anesthesiologists
- Pathologists
- Infectious disease physicians
- Hospitalists
- Intensivists/critical care physicians

Community-based physicians

You can break this group down in several ways to train the largest number of members. First, you may want to meet with the medical leadership group of the medical executive committee to explain the CDI program and how it will be rolled out. After you have spent some time with the medical staff leadership, you will want to focus on education and information sessions for each specialty.

Physicians' should get their first taste of this information at medical specialty meetings. It introduces physicians to the process on their own "territory," so to speak. After this initial introduction by specialty, venture out into the larger physician community to provide sessions for group practices. Further, based on your initial ratings of physicians into one of three categories (leaders/early adopters, late adopters, or non-adopters), target some individuals or small groups for focused information sessions.

Nonphysician clinicians

Generally, the more clinical practitioners you can reach with your CDI message, the more effective the program will be. This does not mean that you should provide the same level of education to every clinician, but it does mean that clinicians should understand the goal of the CDI program when they hear someone speak about it. If a physician has a question, any clinician in the hospital should at least be able to direct the physician to the necessary resource for an answer. Or, if your hospital prides itself on customer service, clinicians should find the answer and give it to the physician. Nonphysician clinicians should all receive general CDI training. Other specific groups, who will be providing ongoing support to the physicians should receive more detailed and focused training. Clinicians who should be included in general training include the following:

- Case managers
- Nurse managers
- Nurses
- Therapists
- Pharmacists
- Central supply technicians
- Utilization review technicians
- Disease management professionals
- Outcomes management professionals
- Quality improvement professionals
- Lab and radiology technicians
- Dietitians

Nonclinical CDI supporters

In addition to the clinical staff addressed above, nonclinical staff also need to play a role (administrative, not clinical) in the educational process. But, again, everyone who is involved in CDI support should be enlisted in basic education. Then, depending on the depth of involvement of each individual or professional area, additional educational sessions should be conducted. At a minimum, individuals from the following areas should be included in initial educational sessions:

- HIM
- Coding
- Case mix
- Reimbursement
- Compliance
- Admitting/registration
- Patient financial services
- Information services

What subjects should the education program include?

Let's look at the content of a general documentation improvement session for clinical and nonclinical personnel. In subsequent chapters, we will address the details that you should include in the sessions focused on clinical or nonclinical groups.

What is a clinical documentation improvement program? (inpatient-specific)

Introduce the concept of CDI by explaining the goals of the program itself, i.e., accurate reimbursement and reliable data.

Clinical documentation improvement is a joint effort between the physicians and the hospital. It ensures that both parties represent the patient's illness and subsequent care as accurately as possible. Include this last concept in your introduction; accuracy is why the program should matter to the clinicians attending.

Reimbursement depends on documentation

Follow the introduction with a reminder that documentation determines the amount of reimbursement that the hospital receives for each inpatient case. In this context, you could use a simplified version of the documentation model we have referred to in previous chapters. It might look something like this:

Physician's documentation → Coding and DRG assignment → Bill to Medicare

A visual rendering of this process will help your audience internalize the concept. Later in the program, reinforce this concept with examples of actual clinical documentation that impacts reimbursement. These examples will help convince clinicians of the need to document the patient's record accurately and completely.

The model above stresses the two most important rules of patient medical record documentation:

1. The attending physician's documentation is key throughout the patient's stay.
2. Documentation is the key to appropriate billing. In each patient's case, documentation forms the basis for coding and the calculation of the bill that shows the cost of the patient's care.

Basics of ICD-9-CM coding assignment (both diagnostic and procedural)

It is important to share some basic concepts of ICD-9-CM assignment in the introductory session because coding determines reimbursement, a main focus of the CDI program. Don't include too much detail in this explanation. Remember, attendees are not there to learn how to code. They are, for the most part, clinicians who can relate best to clinical documentation issues. If you begin to weigh down the process with details about how ICD-9-CM codes are actually assigned, you will lose your students' attention and possibly even their support. You should include a reference to the following concepts:

- Describe the "principal diagnosis" as defined in *Uniform Hospital Discharge Data Set (UHDDS)* guidelines. Your audience should understand that they can assign only one of the patient's conditions as the principal diagnosis. (The patient's condition, established after study, is the one that occasioned the hospital admission.)

- Describe the concept of a "secondary diagnosis" under *UHDDS* guidelines and provide the audience with a copy of the criteria for when it is appropriate to code a secondary diagnosis.

- Explain that a credentialed coding professional assigns an ICD-9-CM code to every diagnosis and every procedure. Coding professionals use official guidelines and current references to translate the physician's documentation into coded data.

As an introduction to your next topic (DRG assignment), explain that ICD-9-CM coding is the basis for DRG assignment. The model will look like this:

Physician documentation → ICD-9-CM coding assignment → DRG assignment → Reimbursement

Basics of DRG assignment

Explain the concept of DRG assignment as well. You can do this through the use of a diagram like the one shown in Figure 5.1.

In the introductory session, you should explain how a code becomes the basis for payment to the hospital. First, the patient's principal diagnosis determines which of the 25 major diagnostic categories (MDCs) clinicians will use. The major diagnostic categories, in general, correspond to the systems in the human body. For example, MDC 1

Figure 5.1 **DRG assignment**

Principal diagnosis assignment

↓

Major diagnostic category assignment (MDC)

↓

Medical vs. surgical designation

↓

Principal procedure (ICD-9-CM code)

↓

Medical vs. surgical DRG designation

↓

DRG assignment

↓

Relative weight x hospital's "blended rate"

↓

Actual reimbursement amount

includes disorders of the nervous system, and MDC 4 includes disorders of the respiratory system. After the patient's case has been assigned to one of the 25 MDCs, it will then be designated as either a medical or surgical case, based on the presence of an operating room (OR) procedure. If an OR procedure is performed, the case is designated as surgical. If not, the case is designated as medical. Finally, based on the diagnostic code and presence of secondary complications or comorbidities, the coder assigns the patient's case a DRG. Each DRG then receives a relative weight. The relative weight is a number from approximately 0.50 to 3.5 that reflects the amount of resources the patient with that set of diagnoses and procedures is likely to consume during his or her stay. The relative weight is then multiplied by the hospital's "blended rate" to determine the exact amount of payment to the hospital. The hospital's blended rate is a specific dollar amount that is assigned to each hospital by the Medicare program. Factors like such as the consumer price index for the region, hospital size and services, and whether the hospital has a teaching component determine the blended rate. For example, congestive heart failure is assigned to DRG 127. Assuming the relative weight for DRG 127 is 1.0110 and ABC Hospital's blended rate is $4,200, the payment for a PPS inpatient with congestive heart failure admitted to ABC Hospital is $4,246.20 (or $4,200 x 1.0110).

Explaining case mix index

Case mix index (CMI), in the inpatient PPS environment, simply means "average relative weight for all PPS patients for a specified period of time." Usually, CMI is calculated in increments of time (e.g., yearly, quarterly, or monthly). Calculations of less than a month are usually not very meaningful. CMI accounts for a large portion of inpatient revenues in most acute care hospitals. A reliable CMI can help predict annual revenues. A hospital can easily project its expected PPS payments for the coming year if it knows, for example, that

- its annual CMI is 1.2895
- it is projecting that it will remain constant for the coming year
- its number of projected PPS patients is 10,000
- its blended rate is $4,200

The process for calculating PPS payments is the following:

CMI × blended rate = Average payment per patient

OR

1.2895 × $4,200 = $5,415.90 (Average payment per patient)

Average payment per patient × expected number of patients in the year = total PPS revenues

OR

$5,415.90 × 10,000 = $54,159,000 (expected annual PPS revenues)

Nonfinancial professionals should remember to always balance revenues against costs. Hospital stand a very good chance of losing money or barely breaking even on most PPS inpatients. It may cost a hospital $55 million to make $54 million providing inpatient care.

Examples of documentation in need of improvement

In your education session, include some examples of cases with potential for documentation improvement that you have found in your own facility. These examples make the process "real," especially to the clinicians. They also show the attendees that there is room for documentation improvement in your organization.

Your role in CDI

Finally, you should end the session with a focus on each individual's role in CDI. This process affects the financial livelihood of the organization; that fact should drive your presentation, and it should motivate everyone to help make this process work. You also should carve out some roles for each of the clinical and nonclinical attendees. We will discuss some of these roles later on in this book.

How to educate

You should ensure that you have the right people delivering the education to your organization. The right message delivered in the wrong manner or by the wrong person can have a negative impact that can be difficult to overcome. This is particularly true when the audience is physicians. For them, make sure your educators are polished professionals who can speak to physicians on their own level. Physicians do not like being "talked down" to, "preached" to, or threatened.

Most important, physicians will not tolerate having their time wasted. The individual conducting these sessions should be able to answer any questions a physician may pose.

When to educate

Proper timing plays an important part in the educational process. Be sure to integrate education with the rest of the CDI program. If, during your session, you mention that clinicians will be on the floors to assist physicians with documentation improvement concerns, but then you don't launch that service for a few months, your program will lose credibility. More important, you may have lost the physicians' willingness to cooperate. Because cooperation is key to the program's success, you should strategically schedule education just prior to, or concurrently with, the rollout of the rest of your program.

CHAPTER 6

Determining Who Will Drive the CDI Process Forward

Determining Who Will Drive the CDI Process Forward

To prepare for the clinical documentation improvement (CDI) process, you need to determine who in your organization will keep things moving. You will need to designate a CDI manager, but documentation improvement takes more than one person or a handful of people. Instead, the program should permeate every department of the facility. Continuity and inclusiveness are the two most important concepts that your organization should focus on when deciding who will drive the CDI process forward.

Multidisciplinary focus

First, let's examine the importance of a multidisciplinary focus. The medical staff has primary authority over clinical documentation for reimbursement purposes. At the same time, every clinician in the healthcare organization should play a role in ensuring that the physician's documentation is accurate. Physicians are already overburdened with patient issues and their own reimbursement concerns, but support from other clinicians can ease that burden. Hospital clinicians in particular should play a role in the CDI program because documentation issues change frequently, and informed clinicians can pass on those changes to physicians.

Involving nonclinical professionals

In addition to nonphysician clinicians, several nonclinical professionals in your organization should also take part in the CDI process. Nonclinical issues often affect documentation. Medicare reimbursement motivates good DRG PPS documentation, so individuals who understand Medicare policy should participate in CDI. These individuals could be HIM professionals, financial professionals, compliance professionals, or other administrators.

Chapter 6

The professionals who participate in the CDI program should come from the following areas:

- Medical staff (community physicians, not employed by the hospital)
- HIM and coding professionals
- Compliance professionals
- Finance professionals
- Case managers
- Nurse managers
- Physician assistants
- Clinicians in the ancillary areas

How can all of these individuals participate in CDI? The beauty of the typical healthcare organization is that most of its functions are integrated: Each one draws upon individuals from multiple specializations.

Think about the typical operating room (OR) procedure. For an operation to succeed, patient registration and admissions staff need to work with the OR scheduling crew to make sure the patient is appropriately scheduled. Then the OR nurse needs to communicate with the surgeon regarding surgical procedures to ensure that central supply sends the correct items, that pharmacy sends the correct drugs, and that any devices that need to be on hand are in the OR. The physician needs to communicate with the anesthesiologist, who in turn needs to communicate with the OR scheduling crew to ensure adequate supplies for anesthesia. At a minimum, the professionals tending to patients during surgery come from anesthesia, surgical specialty, nursing, and pathology. Successful healthcare organizations take this concept of involving various disciplines in a single task and roll carry it out in all areas of the facility. Your organization should incorporate this process in its CDI program as well.

You can involve individuals from various disciplines in several ways. The simplest method is to ensure that any continuing education or information sessions that you plan for CDI include invitations to as many of these professionals as possible. Depending on your organization, you may want designate one or more individuals from each area as CDI contact persons. These people would help communicate CDI developments. You may also want to schedule regular meetings (i.e., quarterly, monthly) during which CDI progress is assessed. Individuals from a variety of disciplines should participate in these meetings. Obtaining participation and feedback from a diverse group ensures that the program does not become flat or ineffective. How your CDI program will take advantage of the many experts who can impact documentation—and hence, reimbursement—depends on the culture of your organization. Figure 6.1 demonstrates some examples of how you can begin to integrate multiple disciplines into your CDI program.

Involving the medical staff

In Chapter 4 we discussed how you might "rate" the physicians on your medical staff as leaders/early adopters, late adopters, and nonadopters. Once you've done that, pull the leaders into your multidisciplinary activities. The more you can involve members of the medical staff in CDI activities, the more successful your program will be. Then, as we discussed before, integrate your late adopters into the CDI program as much as

Figure 6.1 **How to Attain a Multidisciplinary CDI Program**

1. Invite all nonclinical professionals to CDI program updates/educational sessions on an annual or biannual basis.
2. Invite individuals from a variety of disciplines to participate in "Documentation excellence—grand rounds." During these rounds, examine and analyze the documentation provided in various inpatient cases and assess its impact on the hospital.
3. Invite designated individuals from each of the disciplines to documentation break out sessions. In these sessions, attendees split up into teams and review specific inpatient records to spot documentation problems. Have the teams solve the problems and use the information as part of your continuous CDI program.
4. Create a standing committee for the CDI with members from all disciplines. Use the committee to develop policies and assess program progress.
5. Integrate documentation improvement into one or many of the other multidisciplinary functions currently ongoing in the hospital. These could include JCAHO accreditation activities, quality improvement initiatives, or corporate compliance.

possible. This is an important strategy. If you can make converts of some late adopters, your chances of gaining the cooperation of other late adopters and nonadopters will greatly improve.

Continuity

Before you commit yourself and your organization to CDI, you should make certain that your organization wants to pursue an activity that requires an ongoing expenditure of resources to succeed. CDI cannot be guided by an ad hoc committee that disbands a short time after implementation. It is a process that must be supported and driven forward assertively. Certainly, the rewards and benefits of such a program will justify the resources necessary to sustain it. If you want your CDI program to succeed in the long term, you have to accept the concept of continuity.

You have some flexibility in how you implement and drive your CDI program forward. Think about the type of structure that works best in your organization and the type of structure that your medical staff will respect. First, let's look at the structures that you could use to advance the CDI program.

Department

Typically, the department drives functions forward in a hospital. Establishing a CDI department can be a positive move politically. For example, if only the department heads in your organization receive recognition, credibility, and respect from their peers, establishing a CDI department may be your best choice. On the other hand, the people in your organization may perceive the CDI manager as just one more manager among many. In this instance, if you want recognition for a cutting-edge function, creating a department may not be the way to go.

If you have an organizational chart, ask yourself this question before you decide where the CDI function should rest: "Where would we put it in the organization chart, and why?" Pondering this question may help you find the best approach to this challenge. If you need an entire department to advance your cause, that realization will help you create a system that fits with your organization.

For example, are you limiting CDI to inpatient care only? This is the trend in acute care hospitals and healthcare organizations, but CDI can improve reimbursement in every healthcare setting. If your organization plans to roll out documentation improvement into all care areas, you may want to establish this function by department.

Part of another department

In some instances it may be easier and potentially more politically correct to house the CDI function, at least initially, within an already established department. Many organizations house the CDI function in HIM, while others set it up in case management. Certainly the skill set of the manager of the CDI program should be taken into consideration when choosing where to place the program. Your organization's view of documentation improvement will help to determine where the CDI function will best fit.

Regardless of your organization's philosophy regarding documentation improvement, you need a core group of people guiding the process with whose skill sets that include coding, PPS programs, clinical issues, and data analysis. These people, as a group, should perform their tasks regardless of where they are located. More important than location of the group and function is the group's access to senior members of administration and the medical staff in the event of certain undesirable events, and access to management for help in solving problems such as uncooperative clinicians or identification of documentation errors that could place the hospital at significant financial risk.

Part of many departments

You could also incorporate CDI into many departments. This model would probably work best in a larger facility. Many organizations use CDI in their accreditation and quality improvement activities. As long as you have a sufficient number of professionals with coding, clinical, PPS, and data analysis skills in each department, splitting CDI among these departments could work. Best of all, this model puts the responsibility for documentation improvement in the areas where it will be most effective. For example, a multidepartment CDI program might include activities in

- case management (for inpatient activities)
- ED (for ED visits)
- each of the ancillary clinical departments, such as lab and radiology (for diagnostic testing)
- the ambulatory surgery unit (for ambulatory surgery visits)
- the inpatient rehabilitation facility (for inpatient rehabilitation visits)

Depending on the size and breadth of your organization, this list could go on to include many more patient care settings.

Committee

Using committees to propel the CDI program is one of the weaker solutions. It can work if you designate a strong manager and if your organization is small and not very complex. The larger an organization becomes, however, the more difficult it will is to get things accomplished by committee. At the same time, even though a committee usually does not work well for promoting CDI, it could be used as a secondary vehicle, especially if a physician leads it. A CDI committee headed by a leader or early adopter physician can benefit any CDI program.

Interdisciplinary function

As we noted above, you need to ensure that the CDI program receives constant attention from a group of multidisciplinary caregivers, both clinicians and nonclinicians. The most creative organizations can incorporate this concept into a management process that relies on CDI as an interdisciplinary function. This management model would ensure that clinicians and nonclinicians throughout the organization, possibly coordinated by one chief person, drive CDI forward. This model is more fluid than the "part of many departments" model discussed earlier, because it allows for crossover among departments and embraces CDI as an integral part of every function. The typical manager may have difficulty grasping this form of CDI, so as your interdisciplinary CDI manager, you should pick someone with a high energy level, an aptitude for creativity, and a willingness to try new things—someone with an entrepreneurial personality.

Identifying a manager for the CDI process

In every instance, the CDI manager must ensure that the targets for documentation improvement are met and refined on an ongoing basis. The success of your program depends on this individual, so he or she should be someone have a stake in the success of your organization, truly care about the viability of the program and the organization, command the respect of your medical staff, and have strong interpersonal and negotiating skills. Many people in your organization may have some or all of these qualities, but you have to consider one additional characteristic that may narrow the playing field: This individual must have the experience and skills that create immediate credibility.

For example, reimbursement managers in your finance department may meet all of the basic criteria, but it is unlikely that they would have the credibility to drive a CDI program. Physicians may view someone with a background in finance as focusing too much on money, and not enough on patient care. Think about potential credibility when you pick your manager.

A number of professionals could manage the CDI process if they meet the criteria noted above. Some of these individuals include physicians, case managers, HIM coding professionals, and nurse managers. In the following section, we explore the ways each of these professionals could manage CDI.

Physicians

Physicians may already have leadership roles in your organization. If they do, consider adding CDI management to their duties. Placing the CDI process under the direct management of a physician in your organization may give the process more credibility, as long as the physician has the respect of his or her peers. Physicians who have their peers' respect have significant advantages in the CDI role over other managers because they have history with at least some medical staff. They can relate to the issues that physicians address when asked to spend more time on higher-quality documentation. Successful physician managers not only relate to the medical staff and acknowledge extra effort that CDI requires, but they are also willing to work with the medical staff to help the hospital. Even if a physician does not run the CDI process, it may be a good idea to add CDI management to the other activities of senior physician leaders.

Case manager

A case manager oversees the activities of a group of patients concurrently, usually all the patients on one nursing unit. There are many different case manager models in the acute care setting. Most case management programs fall into one of three primary types. The first is the utilization review (UR)/discharge planning model, in which the case manager focuses on insurance approval and UR activities to ensure that the patient's insurance company will pay for his or her stay. In this model, the case manager also manages discharge planning.

Next is the outcomes/disease management model, in which the case manager focuses primarily on clinical activities and disease paths. The third model is a hybrid of the first two models, and the case managers are responsible for both clinical and UR/discharge planning.

Depending on the model employed in your organization, you may want to choose someone with a case management background to head up the CDI program. Case managers who have worked with your physicians on outcomes and disease management may have more positive relationships with the medical staff than those involved in UR/discharge planning alone. In this model, physicians may see the case managers as allies in patient treatment. In the UR model, however, physicians may think that case managers just want to move the patient out of acute care to a lower, less expensive level of care (although this is certainly not the only objective of utilization review).

Consider the case management model that your organization employs when you decide whether someone with case management background should manage the CDI process. Consider as well the medical staff perception of case management in general, and look at the backgrounds of your case managers. Most are registered nurses, and many hold master's degrees. Clinical background is an important consideration in selecting a CDI manager.

HIM coding professional

The credentialed HIM professional has the advantage of being intimately familiar with the reimbursement system itself, or at least with the documentation required. The HIM professional, however, lacks the hands-on clinical experience of the case manager or other nursing professionals.

To be sure, a clinical professional with reimbursement experience is a rare find. But the CDI program needs to have individuals on the team with just such expertise. You'll have to decide whether your CDI manager needs this expertise. Find out whether the HIM professional has had positive relationships with physicians in the past, whether the candidate has the respect of the medical staff, and whether he or she can communicate effectively with physicians regarding clinical issues. While CDI program directors don't make clinical decisions, they have to respond to clinically related questions from physicians.

Nurse manager

The typical nurse manager has a clinical focus and the ability to coordinate staff to ensure high-quality patient care. This initial description might lead you to believe that a nurse manager might make the best CDI manager. But most nurse managers have little to no exposure to reimbursement issues. This lack of experience may or may not hinder nurse managers in their usual capacity, but they have to fill that void quickly if they want to play a role in CDI.

Qualifications of the CDI manager

The CDI function should draw on individuals with skill sets ranging from clinical to reimbursement-oriented, but you need to look for specific qualifications in your CDI manager. Some of those qualifications are described below.

Strong sales skills

For CDI to succeed, you need to sell the program constantly to the members of the medical staff. Above all, the CDI manager needs to realize this necessity. Managers, even physicians, will fail if they expect their fellow physicians to cooperate with a program because the hospital demands it, or if they try to force it on them.

Results oriented

The leader of the program needs to be constantly linking the physicians' activities to data that shows some movement in the right direction. Data analysis isn't just a one-time process that takes place after the initial implementation of CDI to show its success. CDI tracking must take place continuously.

Good negotiator

CDI managers need to constantly negotiate with physicians on behalf of the hospital. The hospital needs the cooperation of the medical staff, and the CDI manager needs to know how to gain that cooperation. Negotiating skills are one of the most useful tools the CDI manager could have.

Excellent public speaker and presenter

On many occasions the CDI manager will need to present information to the medical staff. Physicians need to respect the CDI manager. Excellent public speaking skills can help a CDI manager gain physicians' respect and cooperation. Physicians should look forward to hearing his or her presentations.

CHAPTER 7

Putting CDI Education into Operation

Putting CDI Education into Operation

Introduction

In a previous chapter, we discussed the initial training considerations in your CDI program. In this chapter, we take that concept a step further by discussing the ways in which you can make the educational process operational. The true success of a CDI program depends upon the extent to which clinicians and physicians can internalize new information and put it into practice. We could even go so far as to say that the success of your CDI program rests upon the extent to which you apply adult learning principles to your population (your physicians and nonphysician clinicians). Let's explore some of those principles.

Practical application of theory

In any learning environment, you have to turn theory into practice. To keep it simple, you can provide examples of the theory you are discussing. Or you can also have audience members participate in problem solving, or split them up into small teams to work on problems together. Adult education experts favor this latter technique. Interaction with other adults to arrive at a solution to the same problem is not only an excellent learning process, it also improves workplace efficiency. Let's look at some examples of how we can put the CDI learning process into operation.

The DRG assignment exercise

In this exercise, participants use actual resources to assign a DRG. Any inpatient documentation improvement program needs to cover the concept of DRG assignment. (For this exercise, you can refer to the list of DRGs in the Appendix.) Provide participants with the following list of diagnoses and procedures and have them assign the correct DRG to each one. Then, have them list the payment and the average length of stay (ALOS).

Diagnosis/Procedure	DRG	Payment	ALOS
CVA	14	$5,000	6.1 days
TIA	15	$3,200	3.7 days
TKR	209	$8,600	5.1 days
UTI with a CC	320	$3,700	5.6 days
UTI without a CC	321	$2,400	3.9 days
Septicemia	416	$7,000	8.0 days
Simple pneumonia with a CC	089	$4,600	6.3 days
Complex pneumonia with a CC	079	$7,400	9.3 days

After the participants have identified the payment and ALOS for the DRGs that you have listed, have them calculate the daily payment for each patient. They will need a calculator, but the process is simple. For example, to calculate the daily payment for a patient with septicemia, you need to divide the total payment ($7,000) by the ALOS (eight days); the answer is $875.00. Now, have the class discuss whether they believe that that amount of money would cover a patient's stay in the hospital for septicemia. Point out to them that that $875.00 is the payment if the patient stays for eight days. Next, have them calculate the payment if the patient only stays for only six days ($1167). And if the patient stays for 10 days? Only $700 per day. Stimulate discussion about the payment and how it is possible to contain costs with this system.

Approaching the difficult physician

Every nonphysician clinician hesitates to approach a physician to ask whether some important piece of documentation may be missing from the a patient's record. Engage your group in a role-play exercise in approaching a physician to ask this question—especially a "problematic" physician. Every organization has one—the physician that no one wants to bother for fear that she or he will lash out in anger, or threaten to send his or her patients to a competing hospital. Every organization must balance the costs and benefits of approaching such a physician. In the course of your educational sessions, have the participants role-play this situation. Then, have the them list the best approaches to the problematic physician.

Identifying a clinical opportunity to support a diagnosis

In this exercise, you will need to use examples of actual documentation from a patient record. Have the participants review some discharge summaries (we have provided several cases in the Appendix). You can use the discharge summaries included in this book, or you can use your own progress notes or discharge summary examples from your hospital's records. Have the participants break up into groups of two or three and discuss among themselves possible documentation improvement opportunities, and how they would suggest them to physicians. What questions would they ask? How would they ask them? How might physicians respond, and how would nonphysician clinicians respond to those comments? You should repeat this activity regularly, not just during initial training. It will assist the clinicians in keeping sharp and up to date on new documentation concerns with physicians.

The case-mix index exercise (or, what happens when the physician's newly added documentation changes the DRG)

Using either the information in the exercise above or your own documentation, have small teams of clinicians perform the following tasks:

- Identify the relative weight and payment for each original DRG – and then the relative weight and payment for the DRG with "improved documentation"
- Identify the difference in relative weight and payment.
- Calculate the total difference in relative weight and payment for each of the DRG changes in the discharge summaries
- Calculate the case mix index for the original DRGs
- Calculate the case mix index for the DRGs with improved documentation
- Discuss the differences possible with documentation improvement

Elbow-to-elbow education

To train nonphysician clinicians to identify possible opportunities for improved clinical documentation, pair them up with experts in documentation and coding in an "elbow-to-elbow" review of inpatient medical records on the nursing unit. The review of documentation in the clinician's actual work environment thus benefits from the feedback of documentation experts who guide the learning process. You can implement elbow-to elbow training using the following steps:

Use the daily census to identify all patients for review.

First, identify the resource that will allow you to track all patients for documentation review. This is most commonly the inpatient census, which may be either computerized or in hard copy format, depending on your organization. In any event, the tool should be used so that all cases that are admitted are reviewed.

Conduct reviews by nursing unit.

It is best to conduct documentation reviews by nursing unit for two reasons: First, inpatient census is generally categorized by nursing unit. Second, clinicians performing reviews will most likely be stationed at distinct nursing units. Therefore, documentation by unit will be the most efficient methodology.

Review each patient case initially and record all necessary data elements.

Initially, the process should involve the documentation specialist (usually an HIM coding professional) who reviews inpatient records and shares findings with the clinicians on the unit. Beginning the process like this allows the documentation specialist to get a handle on the overall documentation challenges in the unit and to determine the specific strategy for improvement by unit. In addition, the clinician on the unit usually has other duties—like utilization review, discharge planning, or clinical outcomes—that she or he is responsible for completing. Documentation review is usually a new part of the clinician's job. A strategy like the one described above, where the documentation specialist begins the review process and then shares the information with the clinician, is an effective way to begin the CDI review process.

The initial data elements that should be reviewed and recorded include the following:

- Patient name/medical record number
- Date of admission
- DRG assignment
- Relative weight
- ALOS
- Type of concurrent query (if asked)

Once this information is recorded, and if a concurrent query has been asked of the physician, a second review should occur to determine if the physician has added the necessary documentation. Then additional data elements should be added to the original list; they should include the following:

a. If the physician did not add any additional information, either review the documentation later, or note that no documentation was added in response to the request.

b. If the physician did add documentation, then add the following data elements:

- New DRG
- New relative weight
- Change in relative weight amount
- New length of stay
- Change in length of stay amount

Provide feedback on each case to the unit clinician.

During the initial set of reviews, the documentation specialist should review each change or query the clinician on the nursing unit. This feedback process should continue for a week or two until the clinician becomes more familiar with the process. The length of time may vary by type of nursing unit; for example, in a nursing unit with mostly orthopedic surgery patients, the diversity of patients is not great, so the initial review process may be streamlined. However, in a general med-surg unit with a great diversity of patients, the clinician may need much more time to become familiar with the different types of patient documentation issues.

Begin to incorporate review.

Eventually, the documentation specialist should begin to shift responsibility for the review from the documentation specialist to the unit-based clinician. This transition can be accomplished through the use of side-by-side review. Working with the clinician, the documentation specialist can initially point out documentation concerns in the records. Eventually, the documentation specialist should transfer that task over to the clinician. After two or three weeks, the clinician should be performing the reviews with the documentation specialist providing only the oversight and feedback.

Transfer review to the clinician with regular feedback.

The final stage of putting the CDI review process into operation involves integrating the function into the day-to-day responsibilities of the unit-based clinician. The documentation expert should provide regular feedback, first on a weekly basis, then monthly. Eventually, documentation audits should be performed on a monthly or quarterly basis as a continuous learning opportunity for the clinician.

Shadowing practices

Shadowing is a practice that can be integrated into the physician learning process. It involves the pairing up of a nonphysician clinician/documentation expert with the physician for a day of patient care. It can occur after physicians have been provided with initial classroom training in CDI and understand its basic concepts in both the hospital and office settings. Shadowing is a practical application that can be used effectively with physicians, as opposed to nonphysician clinicians. The documentation expert "shadows" the physician, and at the end of the day, the two practitioners compare notes on what should have been documented based on what the physician did for each patient. This practice involves a lot of feedback from the documentation expert to the physician and can greatly benefit the physician who is open to receiving and using the feedback. Physician shadowing can be implemented using the following steps:

1. Choose appropriate individuals to perform the shadowing.
The selection of appropriate individuals to shadow physicians is an essential element in the success of the program. Those individuals must be able to communicate with the physicians on a clinical level and must also understand the importance of complete and accurate documentation. They must be detail oriented and have excellent investigative skills. Moreover, they must be excellent negotiators and enjoy the respect of the physicians in your organization.

2. Identify physicians willing to participate in the process.
You may have some leaders or early adopters from the list that you developed in a previous chapter. If so, these may be some of the physicians that you will want to approach to participate in the shadow audit process.

3. Test the process with a few select physicians
Once you have identified a few physicians willing to be shadowed, you will want to test the process. Work with a few physicians initially to define your process because shadowing never works exactly in the same way in every organization.

4. Define the method that will work for your organization.
Use the test run to define your process. For example, is shadowing done for a full day or only part of a day in your organization? When can you provide the feedback to the physician being shadowed—right after the patient's been seen, or at the end of the day? What specific information do physicians in your organization want to focus on? Some of these responses will be based on the type of organization and whether physicians are employed at the facility or based in the community.

5. Create a "hook" to persuade physicians to participate in shadowing.
Shadowing is not an activity that can be forced on physicians. In fact, if you are very selective about whom you ask to participate, physicians may actually request that they

be included. The best scenario for your operation is to have physicians come to you and ask for your assistance. The results can be extremely helpful, not only to the organization but also to the physician.

6. Invite other physicians to participate.
Remember that shadowing should not be mandatory for any physicians. They must want to participate. Without their support, the process will not be very valuable. As noted above, you may want to make it known to physicians that the shadowing activity is available to them and that the process involves feedback on documentation that may impact hospital as well as professional reimbursement. You will also want to note that this service is limited, and given the scarcity of individuals who are qualified to shadow the physicians, this will probably be a true statement. In the best-case scenario, physicians will come to you. If they do not, you may want to engage in some additional marketing activities. But chances are that the word of other physicians who have been involved in shadowing will increase demand for the service.

Using surveys and self-assessment instruments

One of the most effective mechanisms to enhance the adult learning process is the self-assessment instrument. In this practice, the adult learner is asked to rate (usually on a scale from 1 to 5) his or her knowledge of subject matter before the educational process as well as after. The greater the difference in ratings between before and after the educational session, the more effective the process. More importantly, this assessment is good evidence of the adult learner's retention. Surveys to collect information on the adult learner's attitudes and opinions about the process may also be employed. While they are not particularly effective in determining the learner's level of retention, surveys can be used for feedback to improve future versions of the sessions. (Please see the self-assessment form at the end of this chapter.)

Self-assessments can be created and implemented using the following steps:

1. Identify all objectives for each learning session.
2. Build the sessions around the specific learning objectives.
3. Create an assessment that requires the participant to address each learning objective separately.
4. On a scale from 1 to 5, have the participant identify his or her knowledge of each objective both before and after the educational sessions.

To determine the effectiveness of the educational sessions based on self –assessments, do the following:

1. Calculate the mean for each objective before and after the educational sessions. Those objectives with higher differences (before to after the learning sessions) indicate the highest learning experiences as a group.
2. Calculate the overall mean (for all objectives) before and after the learning sessions. The closer the mean for after the sessions is to 5, the more effective the sessions have been.

Incorporating post-tests into all educational sessions

A post-test that specifically addresses the objectives of the learning session can be a valuable tool for reinforcing short-term retention. The post-test should contain multiple-choice questions on each of the learning objectives that composed the session. Participants should take the test and receive immediate feedback, which should include explanations of why certain answers were correct. And participants should be encouraged to ask questions and comment on difficult or confusing questions. This information can be used to ensure that the tests, going forward, are fair and consistent. Post-tests should be graded and copies provided to the attendees. Original tests should be retained in the participant's HR folder for some period of time as evidence of the session as well as the participant's initial retention of information. Additionally, you can analyze the test questions by identifying the percentage of test takers who scored correctly or incorrectly on each question. Eventually, the result should be a test that contains equal portions of very difficult, moderately difficult, and mildly difficult questions—a reliable measure of useful information that is being communicated through the sessions. (Please see the sample post-test at the end of this chapter.)

Conclusion

We have discussed several different methodologies to use in CDI educational sessions. The best approach is to incorporate as many of the different methods into your training as you can. For example, in planning a session, show the practical application of theory, have participants interact with one another to solve problems, give them a post-test, and then have them perform a self-assessment to rate their retention of the subject matter.

Figure 7.1

HP3 Healthcare Concepts, Inc
DOCUMENTATION IMPROVEMENT PROGRAM
Case Manager Self-Evaluation

Directions: Please complete the following statements by indicating your level of knowledge and familiarity with the concepts addressed before the start of the documentation improvement program as well as your knowledge currently of the same concepts. Circle the number which best represents your level of knowledge and familiarity both before and currently. "1" signifies no knowledge and "5" represents a strong knowledge of the concept.

My knowledge of:	**Before Training**					**After Training**				
	Weak				Strong	Weak				Strong
1. The relationship between documentation & coding	1	2	3	4	5	1	2	3	4	5
2. The relationship between coding & reimbursement	1	2	3	4	5	1	2	3	4	5
3. General logic of the DRG System	1	2	3	4	5	1	2	3	4	5
4. A patient's principal diagnosis	1	2	3	4	5	1	2	3	4	5
5. The role of secondary diagnoses/CCs	1	2	3	4	5	1	2	3	4	5
6. Case Mix Index (CMI)	1	2	3	4	5	1	2	3	4	5
7. The importance of the physician documenting a patient's condition	1	2	3	4	5	1	2	3	4	5
8. The need for physicians to document the significance of lab/other test results	1	2	3	4	5	1	2	3	4	5
9. How pneumonia is categorized in the DRG system	1	2	3	4	5	1	2	3	4	5
10. The difference between reimbursement for simple (79/80) versus complex pneumonia (89/90)	1	2	3	4	5	1	2	3	4	5
11. The difference between reimbursement for COPD vs. respiratory failure	1	2	3	4	5	1	2	3	4	5

Figure 7.1

HP3 Healthcare Concepts, Inc
DOCUMENTATION IMPROVEMENT PROGRAM
Case Manager Self-Evaluation (continued)

My knowledge of:	Before Training	After Training
12. The difference between reimbursement for septicemia vs. "urosepsis"	1 2 3 4 5	1 2 3 4 5
13. The impact that secondary diagnoses can make on the reimbursement for acute MI patients	1 2 3 4 5	1 2 3 4 5
14. The impact that "complex cardiac conditions" can make on reimbursement for patients with cardiac caths during the current stay	1 2 3 4 5	1 2 3 4 5
15. How to identify "gaps" in physician documentation related to reimbursement (DRG) concepts	1 2 3 4 5	1 2 3 4 5
16. The significant difference in reimbursement for most surgical cases if a secondary diagnosis/CC is present	1 2 3 4 5	1 2 3 4 5
17. The importance of identifying the etiology for symptoms, if known	1 2 3 4 5	1 2 3 4 5
18. The importance of documenting differential diagnoses for symptoms with uncertain etiology	1 2 3 4 5	1 2 3 4 5
19. The reimbursement principle that requires the coding of any condition that a physician documents as "possible" "probable" or "questionable" as though the condition exists	1 2 3 4 5	1 2 3 4 5

I would like to know more about:

Other comments:

Figure 7.2

Clinical Documentation Improvement Program
Case Manager's Training Session

Session Post-Test

That condition established after admission, determined to have caused the patient's admission to the hospital is the patient's:

a. primary diagnosis
b. principal diagnosis
c. complication
d. comorbidity

A patient is admitted with SOB and extreme fatigue. Initial impression was community acquired pneumonia. After CXR, CT scan and additional testing a nodule was found in the patient's lung that was determined to be positive for oat cell CA. Pneumonia was ruled out via culture and sensitivity. What is the patient's principal diagnosis here?

a. SOB and extreme fatigue
b. Community acquired pneumonia
c. Lung nodule
d. Oat cell CA

A patient is admitted for BPH and a TURP. In the patient's H&P the attending physician documents a history of COPD and CHF. In addition, during the patient's stay, the patient develops hematuria that the physician documents in the progress notes. A C&S of the urine revealed >100,000 colonies of e. coli. Patient was placed on unasyn. What are the valid secondary diagnoses for this patient?

a. COPD, CHF, hematuria and UTI
b. COPD, and hematuria
c. COPD and CHF
d. COPD, CHF and hematuria

Figure 7.2

Clinical Documentation Improvement Program Case Manager's Training Session (continued)

What is an example of an MDC under the DRG system?

a. pneumonia
b. respiratory disorders
c. patients >65 years old
d. patients with LOS <30 days

Which of the following is an example of a common complication/comorbidity under the DRG system?

a. hypertension
b. uncomplicated diabetes type II
c. hypokalemia
d. seizure disorder

Which of the following elements can affect the hospital's reimbursement for a Medicare patient?

a. principal diagnosis
b. secondary diagnosis
c. operating room procedure
d. all of the above

A physician documents a patient with a final diagnosis of chest pain. What might you be looking for in the patient's record to provide improvement in this physician's documentation?

a. a complication
b. a comorbidity
c. the cause or possible cause for the chest pain
d. an OR procedure

Figure 7.2

Clinical Documentation Improvement Program
Case Manager's Training Session (continued)

Which of the following diagnoses is a cardiovascular condition under the DRG system – affecting patients with acute MIs?

a. hypertension
b. bradycardia
c. hypotension
d. UTI

Which of the following diagnoses is a complex cardiac conditions affecting patients with cardiac caths performed during their inpatient admission?

a. Hypotension
b. Heart block
c. Tachycardia
d. Pneumonia

Where in the patient's record is the best location for physicians to provide documentation of the patient's diagnoses?

a. discharge summary
b. face sheet
c. progress notes
d. orders

CHAPTER 8

Designing CDI Tools

Designing CDI Tools

Every CDI program should run on tools designed for the organization that will be using them. You can design a set of generic tools and supply them to any healthcare provider, but custom-designed tools are more likely to succeed in your organization. The instruments you use to help your staff get better at documenting their work and their patients' conditions can take many forms. Such documentation aids include the following:

- laminated pocket cards
- templates for history & physical (H&P) exams, progress notes, and other forms
- books, either off-the-shelf or custom-designed
- query forms
- software
- reminders, either posted on the wall or in a patient's record
- videos
- Web-based learning

In this chapter, we will discuss the general concept of tool design and development, the types of CDI tools that you should develop, and who should be involved in their design. We will also address the updating and refinement process.

Tool design is only a small part of your CDI program. If you rely on tools at the expense of physician and clinician interaction and cooperation, your CDI program will likely fail.

What is a CDI tool?

Generally, a CDI tool explains specific pieces or general concepts of the CDI program. Tools can, and should, take the shape that lets users get the most out of them. In creating CDI tools, keep in mind that "if all you have is a hammer, every problem looks like a nail." Therefore, tools should be developed for every possible challenge that may be encountered in the CDI program. This includes any challenges that physicians, nonphysician clinicians, or other staff members may face.

The purpose of CDI tools

The ultimate purpose of CDI tools is to help the user implement the CDI program as effectively as possible. Because the program involves many participants, they'll need to use different tools for different functions. As a whole, the group of tools that you develop should increase the effectiveness of your CDI team. Specifically, CDI tools should serve to assist, refresh, prompt, refine, and promote information.

To assist

Each tool should help the user meet the goals of the CDI program. For example, the neurologist's tool should address the types of patients this physician is most likely to see. The tool should help the neurologist find the correct type of documentation for that specialty.

To refresh

Each tool should contain key bits of information to refresh the user's memory of documentation issues. For example, the case manager's tool should contain lists of common secondary diagnoses that are also considered complications or comorbidities, so that the case manager can determine whether the patient record contains clinical evidence of any of these conditions.

To prompt

Each tool should contain information that directs or prompts the user to focus his or her energies on the documentation concerns most likely to impact overall classification of the patient's case. For example, a listing on each tool of common DRGs by specialty can remind the user of the conditions that require a complication or comorbidity to justify the use of more resources for that patient.

To refine

Each tool should contain some level of detail that can help more experienced users refine their documentation. For example, the case manager's tool should contain information that lists the average length of stay (ALOS) for the patient, based on the DRG into which the patient's case is assigned. This would make the tool more useful for the experienced case manager, who has been applying admission and LOS criteria in his or her utilization role. With this information, the experienced case manager can immediately determine whether the average LOS by DRG is higher or lower than the LOS criteria applied for acute care utilization.

To promote innovation

To the extent possible, your organization should use or develop tools as a continuing source of innovation for the CDI program. For example, the tools should encourage feedback from the users. In addition, it may be possible to leave blank spaces in certain tools that allow the user to create user-defined fields. This allows a review of the user tools to uncover innovative future uses.

Characteristics of CDI tools

There are certain characteristics that all CDI tools should seek to maintain. Some of the more important characteristics include convenience, ease of use, and cost-effectiveness.

Convenience

Convenience can mean that the tools are easily placed at nursing units, in one's pocket, or in other easy-to-reach places. Organizations may decide that the tools should be placed in each patient record or be available at every physician dictation station. You could also place documentation improvement tools in the physician's lounge.

Ease of use

For ease of use, tools may be color-coded or set in large print (for easy reading). The size and form of the tool should conform to the needs of the user.

Cost-effectiveness

The cost of development and reproduction should be considered in the design process. Designing a tool that cannot be reproduced economically wastes hospital resources. See how much money you can budget for documentation improvement tools before the process begins. At the same time, encourage participants to "think out of the box." Document even the costliest ideas for possible future inclusion. Then, focus on the tools that fit into your budgetary allowance.

Types of CDI tools

Pocket tools

Pocket tools are generally printed instructions for documenting certain conditions, specialties, and procedures, and they come in a small or pocket-sized format. Generally, physicians and clinicians should carry these with them. They should be printed on durable material, such as plastic or laminated paper. They should also be printed in large quantities so that they can be redistributed and kept in common areas of the hospital, such as the dictation stations, for physicians to pick up on an as-needed basis. Figure 8.1 shows an example of a pocket tool.

Figure 8.1 **Cardiology Doc Pocket Tool titled Common Cardiology DRGs**

CARDIOLOGY
DOC POCKET TOOL

Common Cardiology DRGs

DRG	Avg. Relative Weight	GLOS
MI w/ comorbidity (121)	1.58	5.6
Cardiac cath w/ comorbidity (124)	1.41	3.6
Cardiac cath w/o comorbidity (125)	1.04	2.2
MI w/o comorbidity (122)	1.02	3.2
CHF (127)	1.01	4.5
Vascular disorders w/ comorbidity (130)	0.94	5.0
Arrhythmia w/ comorbidity (138)	0.82	3.3
Thrombophlebitis (128)	0.73	5.2
Syncope w/ comorbidity (141)	0.72	3.0
Vascular disorders w/o comorbidity (131)	0.57	3.8
Syncope w/o comorbidity (142)	0.54	2.2
Angina (140)	0.53	2.2
Chest pain (143)	0.52	1.7
Arrhythmia w/o comorbidity (139)	0.50	2.1

Acute MI Patients – Common Comorbidities

Please document, if present, the conditions listed below for MI patients

- Acute renal failure
- ARDS
- Atelectasis
- Atrial fibrillation
- CHF
- Hypotension
- LBBB
- Paroxysmal SVT
- Ventricular tachycardia
- Respiratory failure
- Trifascicular block
- Ventricular fibrillation/flutter

Patients with Cardiac Cath During this Admission without AMI

Please document, if present, the conditions listed below for cath patients:

- Unstable angina
- CHF
- Cardiac arrest
- Cardiomyopathy
- Endocarditis
- Myocarditis
- Tachycardia

Figure 8.1 **Cardiology Doc Pocket Tool titled Comorbidities/Secondary Conditions**

CARDIOLOGY
DOC POCKET TOOL

Comorbidities/Secondary Conditions

Please document the following secondary conditions, if present, for all types of patients. Conditions shall only be documented if they meet one of the following criteria. The condition was:

1. Clinically evaluated during the stay; or
2. Diagnostically tested during the stay; or
3. Therapeutically treated during the stay; or
4. Increased LOS or nursing care/monitoring

Common Comorbidities/Secondary Conditions

Angina	Diabetes, Type I	Mitral valve prolapse
Atrial fibrillation	Diabetes, uncontrolled	Renal failure, chronic or acute
Anemia, blood loss	Decubitus ulcer	Respiratory failure
Atelectasis	Dehydration	Seizures
Cardiomyopathy	Hyponatremia	UTI
COPD	Ileus	Urinary retention
CHF	Malnutrition	
Cirrhosis		

Symptoms

For patients admitted with symptoms, please document conditions that you are "ruling out". It is helpful to document "differential diagnoses". Conditions documented as possible, probable, rule out or questionable are coded in the inpatient setting only.

Tests

Whenever you order a test, document the "reason" for the test in the progress notes or your orders. (e.g., H/H for weakness, rule out blood loss anemia) Include BOTH the symptom and the condition that you are attempting to rule out.

Whenever tests are abnormal, document the condition that the abnormal result represents. (e.g., for a low sodium – document "hyponatremia" if it exists)

Templates

Templates are guidelines that are printed directly on an 8.5″ x 11″ piece of paper. They instruct physicians about the level of detail or specific information that they should include in a patient's progress note or report. Many hospitals use templates for H&P exams. These templates can be streamlined or redesigned to include hospital CDI concepts. Generally, for CDI purposes, progress note templates are the most useful documentation aid. Templates should contain both hospital CDI as well as physician-office CDI guidelines. Templates can help physicians improve their documentation, which should motivate the medical staff to use them. See Figure 8.2 for a sample template.

Book resources

Book resources can be purchased or designed specifically for use by physicians or clinicians. You can easily create books that contain useful information, such as a listing of DRGs with relative weights, from publicly available files. See Figure 8.3 for a list of

Figure 8.2

Sample Hospital Inpatient Hospital Care

Date ____/____/____

Physical Examination	Temp	BP	Pulse	RR	WT	HT

	Normal	Abnormal (Include pertinent findings)
Constitutional	❐	
Eyes	❐	
ENMT	❐	
Cardiovascular	❐	
Respiratory	❐	
GI	❐	
GU	❐	
Musculoskeletal	❐	
Integumentary (skin, breast)	❐	
Neurologic	❐	
Psychiatric	❐	
Hem/Lymph	❐	

PHYSICAL EXAM

Tests/Radiology	Normal	If abnormal, document specific diagnoses
CBC	❐	
WBC	❐	
Hgb/HCT	❐	
Urinalysis	❐	
Sputum Culture	❐	
Blood Culture	❐	
Blood Gases	❐	
Electrolyte Panel	❐	
Toxicology	❐	
Other Labs (please specify)	❐	
X-ray	❐	
MRI	❐	
Echocardiogram	❐	
EKG	❐	
CT-Scan	❐	
Ultrasound	❐	
Other Radiology (please specify)	❐	

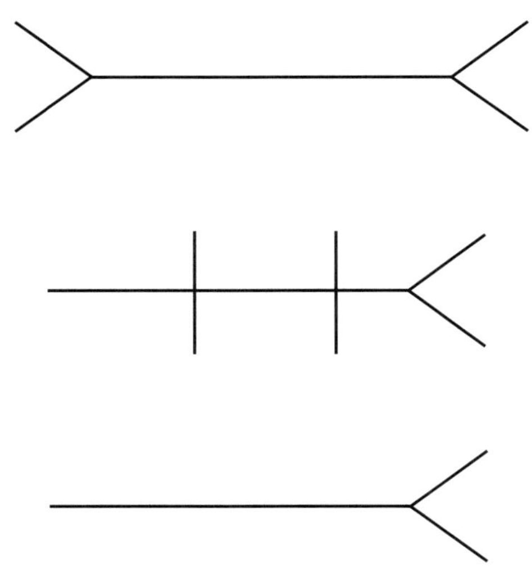

LABS/RADIOLOGY

Figure 8.2

Sample Hospital Inpatient Hospital Care (continued)

Differential diagnoses (for symptoms): ____________________

Secondary diagnoses:

❐ angina ________ ❐ atrial fibrillation ________ ❐ aortic valve disorder ________

❐ cardiomyopathy ________ ❐ CHF ________ ❐ mitral valve prolapse ________

❐ seizures ________ ❐ COPD ________ ❐ dehydration ________

❐ ileus ________ ❐ malnutrition ________ ❐ decubitus ulcer ________

❐ renal failure ________ ❐ diabetes, uncontrolled ________

❐ diabetes w/vascular manifestation ____________________

❐ diabetes w/renal manifestation ____________________

❐ diabetes w/neurological manifestation ____________________

other: ____________________

Assessment/Plan: ____________________

____

Signature: ________________ Date: ________________

GENERAL PROGRESS NOTE TEMPLATE

DRGs with relative weights. (See the Appendix for the full version of the DRG weight chart) In addition, during the product development process, you can customize books to the needs of your organization. For example, you may want to create a small book with DRG information by specialty for orthopedic surgery specialists. You would provide them only with DRG, relative weight, reimbursement, and LOS information for orthopedic surgery DRGs.

Query forms: Paper format

Case managers or nonphysician clinicians use query forms to communicate with the physician. With these forms, case managers or clinicians collect clinical information from the patient's record, and based on that information they ask the physician to clarify documentation in the patient's record. Query forms are important to the CDI program, as they may be the key to either concurrent or retrospective communication with the physician. The forms should not lead the physician, and they should include documentation about clinical factors in the actual record. The following question would be an example of a leading query for a patient with pneumonia: "Does this patient have aspiration pneumonia?" Rephrasing that question in a nonleading format might sound something like this: "Based on the results of the following study, can you

Figure 8.3

DRG Weights

DRG WEIGHTS

DRG	DRG Name	Weight
001	CRANIOTOMY AGE >17 EXCEPT FOR TRAUMA	3.2713
002	CRANIOTOMY FOR TRAUMA AGE >17	3.3874
003	CRANIOTOMY AGE 0-17	1.9594
004	SPINAL PROCEDURES	2.4148
005	EXTRACRANIAL VASCULAR PROCEDURES	1.3628
006	CARPAL TUNNEL RELEASE	0.7230
007	PERIPH & CRANIAL NERVE & OTHER NERV SYST PROC W CC	2.6285
008	PERIPH & CRANIAL NERVE & OTHER NERV SYST PROC W/O CC	1.3953
009	SPINAL DISORDERS & INJURIES	1.3350
010	NERVOUS SYSTEM NEOPLASMS W CC	1.2690
011	NERVOUS SYSTEM NEOPLASMS W/O CC	0.8471
012	DEGENERATIVE NERVOUS SYSTEM DISORDERS	0.9020
013	MULTIPLE SCLEROSIS & CEREBELLAR ATAXIA	0.8129
014	SPECIFIC CEREBROVASCULAR DISORDERS EXCEPT TIA	1.1655
015	TRANSIENT ISCHEMIC ATTACK & PRECEREBRAL OCCLUSIONS	0.7349
016	NONSPECIFIC CEREBROVASCULAR DISORDERS W CC	1.1867
017	NONSPECIFIC CEREBROVASCULAR DISORDERS W/O CC	0.6689
018	CRANIAL & PERIPHERAL NERVE DISORDERS W CC	0.9744
019	CRANIAL & PERIPHERAL NERVE DISORDERS W/O CC	0.6756
020	NERVOUS SYSTEM INFECTION EXCEPT VIRAL MENINGITIS	2.7764
021	VIRAL MENINGITIS	1.4573
022	HYPERTENSIVE ENCEPHALOPATHY	1.0037
023	NONTRAUMATIC STUPOR & COMA	0.8069
024	SEIZURE & HEADACHE AGE >17 W CC	1.0172
025	SEIZURE & HEADACHE AGE >17 W/O CC	0.5947
026	SEIZURE & HEADACHE AGE 0-17	0.5981
027	TRAUMATIC STUPOR & COMA, COMA >1 HR	1.3514
028	TRAUMATIC STUPOR & COMA, COMA <1 HR AGE >17 W CC	1.3609
029	TRAUMATIC STUPOR & COMA, COMA <1 HR AGE >17 W/O CC	0.6956

identify the specific type of pneumonia this patient has?" A sample query form in paper format is shown in Figure 8.4.

Query forms: Stick-on notes

Stick-on notes are an innovative tool for querying a physician. Essentially, you can design mini-query forms that fit onto stick-on notes and place them in the patient's record during the stay. The stick-on notes should instruct the physician to document any additional information in the record. See Figure 8.5 for a sample stick-on query form. Stick-on notes should be used according to the same guidelines as any other query form. If you use them, however, the physician may not document on the stick-on note, and the note may not be made a permanent part of the patient record.

Computer programs with flags

In some instances, you may be able to take advantage of existing computer programs for documentation improvement. For example, case management software may have some applications that allow you to flag certain diagnoses. If you use this kind of software, you may want to flag admitting diagnoses that need a specific query form or stick-on note to communicate with the physician as soon as the patient is admitted.

Personal digital assistant (PDA) applications

You may be able to build personal digital assistant (PDA) applications that are similar to other computer programs (brand names for these devices include Palm Pilot, Visor, and Blackberry). For example, PDA applications that allow physicians or clinicians to identify a working DRG upon admission can be useful. You will need to determine if your budget can handle the increased costs of most automated applications like computer programs and PDA applications.

Posted signs

Although it may sound simplistic, posting signs with important documentation points can help the CDI initiative. Posting signs can supplement other tools. For example, you may want to post a note in the physician dictation area that stresses the importance of documenting secondary diagnoses.

Temporary record forms

You can also place smaller versions of the signs discussed above in patient records as a way of reminding the physician of certain documentation concerns. It will reinforce these concerns if the physician sees the notes both at the dictation stations as well as in the patient records.

Figure 8.4

County Hospital
Pneumonia Query Form

THANKS IN ADVANCE FOR YOUR HELP IN ENSURING ACCURATE DATA FOR THE HOSPITAL!

Patient name: ____________________ MR#: _________ Discharge Date: _________

Dear Dr. _________________________:

Re: Your diagnosis of pneumonia on this patient

Based on the following documentation:

[] positive culture and sensitivity _________________
[] positive lab report of_________________________
[] other report findings:________________________
[] treatment with______________________________
[] other:_____________________________________

There is evidence that you are definitively or possibly treating a specific organism or type of pneumonia. We would like you to provide clarification of your documentation so we can code this diagnosis appropriately. Please specify below the organism or type of pneumonia you are treating:

[] unspecified pneumonia [] viral pneumonia	[] gram negative: Circle one	[] gram positive Circle one	[] other: Circle one
	Klebsiella species	Staph aureus	Aspiration
	Proteus mirabilis	MRSA	Mycoplasma
	Pseudomonas	Streptococcus pneumoniae	Clamydia
	E-coli	Other gram pos:_________	Candida
	Legionella		other:_____
	Hemophilus influenzae		
	Actinobacter		
	Enterobacter		
	Serratia		
	Other gram negative:_________		

Your comments:

If you have questions, please contact the HIM Department at extension ___________

Please sign and date.

Physician signature:_______________________________________ **Date:**_________________

Coder/reviewer name & credentials: _________________________ **Date:**_________________

In the interest of saving you time in the future, more detailed documentation and explanations containing the actual organism you are treating or the organism you believe you are treating will allow us to code correctly without your intervention retrospectively. Thank you!

Figure 8.5 **Respiratory Failure?**

Dear Dr. ________________: Date: _________

Based on clinical criteria this patient meets the definition of respiratory failure. If the patient has respiratory failure, please document it clearly in the progress notes.

Clinical criteria:

PaO2 <60 mmHg and/or PaCO2>50 mmHg

and

pH <7.35

RESPIRATORY FAILURE ?

Document these findings in the record

Doc Notes™ ©2002 HP3 Healthcare Concepts, Inc.

For example, you may want to adopt a practice of placing a CDI form on the records of all patients who are admitted with only a symptom for a principal diagnosis. This form would instruct the physician to identify the potential causes or conditions that are being worked up to identify the etiology of the symptom. For example, a physician may admit a patient for syncope and document the patient's condition as such. However, during the stay the physician may order a CT Scan and an MRI to rule out a CVA, and an echocardiogram and an EKG to rule out arrhythmia or CHF. In other words, the physician should be documenting both the fact that the patient presented with "syncope" and the fact that the patient was worked up for CVA and arrhythmia. From a complete and compliant documentation perspective, the physician must also document when and if the CVA or arrhythmia have been either confirmed or ruled out.

Videos

Videos can serve as an educational tool that continuously reinforces the CDI program. The following list presents the pros and cons of video training:

Video training

Advantages:

- Consistent in delivery of content
- Able to be replayed in portions for clarification of content
- Cost- effective
- Convenient—employees can be trained anytime, anywhere

Disadvantages:

- Interactivity using the video alone is limited
- Unless professionally produced, delivery may be flat and boring
- Specialized equipment is needed

Methods of increasing interactivity:

- Have a training coordinator present to stop the videos at varying points and discuss issues with the trainees/viewers.
- Have the training coordinator available to answer trainee questions throughout the viewing period.
- Conduct training sessions with groups of employees to increase interactivity among participants.
- Conduct a pre- and post- test and provide answers to the tests at the end of the session.
- Create a work book that trainees can use to record pertinent information.
- Use videos that are entertaining enough to hold the attention of the trainee.

Web-based learning

All staff, physicians, clinicians, and nonclinical staff can use Web-based learning to reinforce their knowledge of certain concepts. This type of educational tool works well with physicians if you also offer continuing medical education to the medical staff.

The custom-designing process

The basic tenet of product development is functionality and user-friendliness. You can ensure that the tools you develop are functional and user-friendly only if you involve the user in developing them. There is no substitute for having the user involved in design, testing, and ongoing retesting of the tool. While you may not have the resources to develop tools according to strict production development guidelines, you should employ the following basic rules to ensure that your tools are effective and accepted:

- Involve the user from the initial stages.
- Be selective with your users.
- Create many prototypes based on user feedback.
- Refine prototypes after users have tried out the product.
- Conduct a formal pilot process (expand the user base).
- Introduce your product using a specific marketing strategy
- Use a specific marketing strategy to introduce your product.<H2

Involve the user from the initial stages

Creating a product without involving the user is like playing a baseball game with your eyes shut. You can do it, but the results are likely to be disastrous. The user should be part of the process from the beginning, because you will get your most functional ideas from users. However, keep in mind that you need to have a non-user product team in place to drive the process forward. Your product team will be responsible for keeping to a schedule, providing an objective point of view, applying a cost-benefit analysis to the process, and ultimately delivering the product on time and on budget.

Be selective with your users

Physicians and case managers will use your tools, but that doesn't mean that just any physician or case manager should be on your product development team. You need to select individuals who are willing to spend the time, provide lots of feedback, and work well in a team environment.

Create many prototypes based on user feedback

Your non-user product team should take copious notes of interviews conducted with users and discussions held with the user team. Note taking, information gathering, and observations should feed into the initial process of creating prototypes. A prototype provides an example of a tool that could be used, and it should be the actual tool, a sketch of the tool, or other example or description of the potential tool. The team will need to vote on which prototypes should be designed initially. You should design more than one prototype for comparative purposes.

Refine prototypes after users have tried out the product

Let your physicians and clinicians use several copies of the prototypes. Then, after the users have tried out the prototypes, gather additional information to determine what types of refinements are needed. Continue to refine and redeploy the prototypes into the field until the product(s) are functional and user-friendly.

Conduct a formal pilot process (expand the user base)

Once you have designed the initial tools, pilot-test them in the field in as many places as possible. Conduct feedback from the users via a survey, and use the feedback for final refinements.

Use a marketing strategy Introduce to introduce your product using a marketing strategy

As with any successful product, you will need to use marketing techniques to introduce the tools to your customers. The strategy may involve a session for all physicians (with dinner served) where you discuss documentation for evaluation and management services and professional fees, as well as hospital documentation. Then introduce your tools. Better yet, have a few physicians who assisted in the design process introduce the tools.

Sample tools

For your reference, here's a list of the sample tools we've provided throughout this chapter:

- Retrospective query forms
- Secondary diagnosis pocket tool—generic
- Principal diagnosis pocket tool—generic
- Clinician reference tool for assigning working DRGs (DRG listing)
- Pocket tools by specialty—nephrology
- One-page physician reminders

CHAPTER 9

Implementing a CDI Process Concurrently

Implementing a CDI Process Concurrently

Concurrent record review is the glue that holds all the pieces of the CDI puzzle together. We'll examine the strengths and weaknesses of several concurrent review models in this chapter. Keep in mind that your CDI program will be more successful if you approach it from several directions. The more places in which your CDI program and the people involved with the program have a presence the greater your chances are of seeing a positive return on your investment—in both accurate reimbursement and data quality. In this chapter, we will discuss the different CDI models to choose from. In addition, we will look at the possibility that job-redesign may be necessary if your program to succeed.

Selecting the model

You will need to select the appropriate participants to roll out the CDI program in your organization. Think through the practical aspects: *Who* will manage concurrent review and physician prompting, and *why* would the identified group want to take on a new task? Whenever you ask people to perform a new task, they automatically wonder (silently or aloud), "What's in it for me?" It's always best to provide that information up front. Here are some of the concepts you will need to think through to prepare for a concurrent CDI review:

- Budget constraints
- Current workload of the target group
- Support of the group manager

Budget constraints

Any additional or hidden costs must be identified up front. If you are planning to roll out the CDI program with internal staff, you will need to identify the trainer, the trainees, and the amount of time it will take to adequately prepare

Chapter 9

the staff for the task of concurrent CDI review. For a single system, medium-sized hospital the program will take six to eight weeks of intensive roll out time. To give yourself a rough estimate of your staff costs, multiply these hours by the hourly rate to replace your internal staff while they are training in order. In addition, you will want to add the costs of tool development, discussed in the previous chapter.

Current workload of the target group

You need to consider the current workload of the target group in the assessment process. For example, if you have identified the case managers to manage concurrent CDI, but the group has recently lost three full-time employees and was understaffed to begin with, this group might not be the best option at this time. In this case, you need to ask yourself what other options exist. Or can you wait to kick off the CDI process until case management staffing has improved?

Support of the group manager

If someone other than you manages the group selected to implement concurrent CDI, then you need to determine whether the group's manager supports this project. Often, higher-level officials order a unit to implement CDI (i.e., the chief executive officer or the chief financial officer) without consulting the group's immediate manager. We all like to think individuals would do what is in the best interest of the organization, but this is not always the case. If you do not have the support of the group's manager, then try to find a way to gain that support. This may be difficult, but working towards a worthwhile goal should provide you with the energy and drive to figure out how to make the program work. The goal, keep in mind, is accurate reimbursement, improve physician relations, better data quality, and all of accompanying advantages.

CDI is a change process

Clinical documentation is not a new concept in any healthcare organization, but for many providers, CDI is. The improvement process can shake up your physicians and anyone else who documents care, not to mention the health care organization itself. Concurrent review is truly a change process, more so than any other component of CDI. For that reason, you should familiarize yourself with the concepts of change management.

People are creatures of habit. Any change can disrupt our neatly structured world and make us feel insecure and out of control. In *Everyone's a Coach* (Zondervan, June

1995), authors Ken Blanchard and Don Shula discuss the seven factors for success in making change happen. You should review these factors and consider their importance to the success of your concurrent CDI review process. The seven key factors are:

1. Leading change (who is responsible)
2. Creating a shared need (why we need to do it)
3. Shaping a vision (what it will look like when we are done)
4. Mobilizing commitment (who else needs to be involved)
5. Modifying systems and structures (how it will fit into the organization)
6. Monitoring progress (how it will be measured)
7. Making it last (how it will get started and last)

In *Management of Organizational Behavior* (Prentice Hall, 2000), Blanchard and co-author Paul Hersey discuss the four levels of support and direction managers need to provide to teams undergoing a "change." They do this with their "situational leadership model," which states that effective leaders adjust their style to provide what the group cannot provide for itself during the period of change. The manager needs to oscillate between closely controlling the CDI team or allowing the team to collaborate on its own.

Training the target group

First, you need a training team

Before you can begin training your target group to roll out concurrent CDI review, you need to select your training team. You should ensure that the core members of your training team possess two qualities: consultative talent and expert technical skill.

Consultative talent

The members of your CDI team must have the ability to act as consultants within your organization. They must be able to view the process as objectively as possible and not get bogged down in day to day issues or pettiness. This is a level of professionalism that is absolutely necessary for the success of the program. In addition, your team members should possess other skills commonly found in a consultative personality, including the ability to treat your trainees like customers, the ability to sell the importance of the CDI program, and the ability to empathize with the target group as they go through the change process.

Technical skill

Expertise in documentation is also a prerequisite for membership on the CDI training team. In addition to inpatient documentation expertise, at least one member of your team should be familiar with physician professional fee coding. Expertise in physician coding and documentation is invaluable in winning doctors over to your side during the CDI process. Missing this one element can mean the difference between the success and failure of your program.

Then, you need "trainees"

The trainees, of course, are the people who will be rolling out the concurrent CDI process and should be very comfortable interacting with physicians and vice versa. Trainees should also have familiarity with patient record content and have some clinical background. You may have other criteria that you want to build into this group. Some organizations want to see nurses or a physician or two on the trainee team. The reality is that your team should not be merely accepted, but welcomed by the medical staff. If you have selected a group that makes physicians cringe, then you probably need to go back to the drawing board and plot a more effective strategy.

Possible groups to implement the concurrent CDI process

Case management model

Case management, or medical management, as the function is becoming increasingly known, is a fairly popular group for implementation of concurrent CDI review. On the positive side, case managers review patient records on the nursing unit concurrently as part of their base job, and they are clinicians who interact with physicians on a regular basis. Most likely, they can digest large amounts of information about clinical conditions and documentation quickly. On the negative side, case managers are usually extremely overworked and are pulled in many directions every day by multiple groups, including insurance companies, patient families, and nursing homes. Because of this, if you target case management as your concurrent CDI group, you will need to analyze workflow and determine how many additional staff will be needed to perform the reviews. If case managers are the only review group, then you will most likely need to plan for at least one to two additional staff members. Finally, depending on your organization, case managers may or may not be esteemed in the eyes of the medical staff. In some instances, case managers are seen as clinical partners with the doctors. In others, physicians run the other way when they see the case managers coming for fear of a demand to discharge a patient.

Hospitalists model

Hospitalists are physicians (usually internal medicine specialists) employed by the hospital to provide care to inpatients. Many hospitals have found that hospitalists can manage the medical needs of both medicine and surgical patients more efficiently than independent physicians. In addition, hospitals can exercise a significant amount of control over hospitalists because these physicians are employees of the hospital. Most hospitals employ only a few, usually four to six, to provide these services. For this reason, it is difficult to imagine hospitalists being solely responsible for the concurrent CDI review. More importantly, given their high salaries, using them for a significant amount of CDI review time may not be justified. However, it is hard to imagine a more perfect group to speak with physicians about their documentation than another group of physicians.

RN documentation specialists model

You would do well to hire and train RN documentation specialists as part of the CDI process. Most facilities do not now employ RNs with documentation training, although RNs in utilization review, quality assurance, or risk management functions may be good recruits. The biggest disadvantage of using RNs for documentation review is that you will need to create and develop this group from scratch. On the plus side, the issue of "change management" for these folks is basically non-existent. Like case managers, they can learn clinical documentation quickly and easily; unlike case managers, they don't have an adversarial relationship with physicians.

Concurrent coding model

Since the onset of the prospective payment system, the popularity of concurrent coding has been cyclical. Concurrent coding was popular in the mid-1980s, decreased in popularity in the late 1980s, became popular again in the early 1990s, and then decreased in popularity again in the late 1990s. Hospitals make the decision to implement concurrent coding, with coders on the nursing units providing concurrent review of the records. Then, after some attrition and no return on investment, hospitals pull the programs. In another five or six years, they may give the concurrent coding process another try. Inevitably, the programs fall apart for a variety of reasons. First, concurrent coding alone requires a higher number of coders than retrospective coding. When the additional function of physician querying is added, hospitals need additional coding staff. In addition, being on the nursing unit significantly increases the stress level of the coder, and many coders are in the profession because they do not want to be in a "treating" profession. This results in a turnover of staff who are very difficult to replace. On the positive side, if you are able to identify a group of coders who can effectively perform concurrent coding and CDI review, inpatient records will not only be coded accurately, but in the most timely manner possible—potentially by the day of discharge!

A hybrid model

You may want to consider combining the models we have addressed above. Realistically, it may be the best way for you to engage the variety of people necessary to make a difference. It may be hard to assemble a core group made up, for example, of some hospitalists, some case managers, and one documentation specialist, but it will probably be worth the extra coordination effort you will expend. A hybrid model might look like this:

1. All players are trained on the CDI process
2. One documentation improvement specialist is primarily responsible for reviewing each record upon admission and placing initial queries based upon clinical evidence in the record
3. Case managers follow up on queries in their units
4. Hospitalists are called in to settle disputes or deal with particularly difficult physicians

This is just one example of a hybrid model that could function well. Of course, the ultimate test is your organization's culture and acceptance of such a model. You need to ensure that you are implementing a system that is a good cultural fit for your organization.

Is job redesign necessary?

Depending on the type of model that you implement for CDI review, the question of job redesign may be a concept that you may or may not need to address. You will need to address job redesign if concurrent coding is your model. In this case, coders will need to add to their job the additional function of concurrently querying physicians on a regular basis to make sure that only correct information gets into the patient's record. In order to ensure an efficient process, you will need to work with the coding staff to identify the best process for incorporation of additional activities. The same will be true for the case manager model. Even if the case manager is used within the hybrid model, as discussed above, there will be a need for some level of job redesign. Someone with operational expertise may be helpful in assisting with the job redesign process. While you need a leader to initially direct the process, the most successful job redesigns inevitably occur when the staff members themselves participate in the process as well.

The implementation process

A project is defined as an activity that has specific beginning and ending points. Because the CDI training has a beginning and an end, it can be considered a project. You should differentiate one-time CDI training from the CDI process itself, which, once implemented, should be ongoing. You will need to identify all of the components of your project along with their time frames. Figure 9.1 shows an example of a training matrix. In addition, a Gantt Chart (Figure 9.2) can help everyone involved in the project. While you may use the chart for managing the project, the trainees can also use the chart to track progress.

Gantt chart: a graphic bar chart that shows the relationship between work planned and completed on one axis and time elapsed on the other. Mechanism devised by Henry Gantt, who also devised an incentive system that gave workers a bonus for completing their jobs in less time than the allowed standard.

Figure 9.1

Sample Training Matrix

Group	Topic	No. of Sessions	Comments
Medical staff, general	Professional Fee CDI	1	Bring tools/samples
Medical staff, medicine group	Use of Templates	3	Sample templates, develop new version
Medical staff, surgeons	Use of Templates	2	Sample templates, develop new version
Case managers	Basic Documentation & DRG Concepts	2	
	Principal Diagnosis Documentation	2	
	Secondary Diagnosis Documentation	3	Begin tool development sessions
	Pulmonary Medicine Documentation	2	
	GI & Nephrology Documentation	2	
	Cardiology Documentation	3	
	Orthopedic Documentation	1	
Coding staff	Querying Physicians	2	Bring sample query forms—develop new
	Understanding the Case Management Job & Focus	2	Plan joint meeting of CM/coding staffs after sessions

Figure 9.2 Sample Hospital CDI Program Plan

Sample Hospital CDI Program Plan

Week	1	2	3	4	5	6	7	8	9	10	11	12	13	14	15	16	17	Notes
Activities (# = completed, 0 = Milestone)																		
Clinical Documentation Improvement Program																		
1. Conduct concurrent record reviews																		
Design interview framework/guide																		
Assign three reviewers per day for three months																		
Organize results into training/operating material for physicians and staff																		
Establish performance measurement system to measure documentation and coding results – current vs. corrected, during the project and ongoing																		
2. Support and educate coding staff																		
Hold educational sessions with specialties																		
Create/distribute pocket guides and other prompting tools																		
3. Support and educate medical staff																		
Hold educational sessions with specialties																		
Create/distribute pocket guides and other prompting tools																		
Meet individually with physicians																		
4. Support and educate case management, utilization review and other staff																		
5. Define structure and systems to maintain documentation improvements on ongoing basis																		

Developing concurrent tracking mechanisms

After the team has been identified and trained, they will need tracking mechanisms to track their work. Your tracking mechanisms should be thorough enough to identify all of the elements necessary to evaluate the success of the program. They should also be simple enough not to overburden the CDI team. We have included sample tracking forms in Figure 9.3.

Figure 9.3a

Documentation Improvement Reports

Documentation Improvement Reports
Query by Employee

Report Date: 1/23/02
Date Range: 01/01/01 to 01/01/03

Employee	Total Queries	# CCs	% CCs	# PDXs	% PDXs	# Positve Response	% Positve Response
Jones Julie	3	3	100.00%			2	66.67%

Figure 9.3b **Documentation Improvement Reports**

Documentation Improvement Reports
Query by Physician

Report Date: 1/23/02
Date Range: 01/01/01 to 01/01/03

Physician	Total Queries	# CCs	% CCs	# PDXs	% PDXs	# Positve Response	% Positve Response
Green, Mike	2	2	100.00%			1	50.00%
Maloy, Chris	1	1	100.00%			1	100.00%

Figure 9.3c **Documentation Improvement Reports**

Documentation Improvement Reports
Query by Unit

Report Date: 1/23/02
Date Range: 01/01/01 to 01/01/03

Unit	Total Queries	# CCs	% CCs	# PDXs	% PDXs	# Positve Response	% Positve Response
2A	3	3	100.00%			2	66.67%

Figure 9.3d

Documentation Improvement Reports

Documentation Improvement Reports
Query Summary

Report Date: 1/23/02
Date Range: 01/01/01 to 01/01/03

Query Type	Count	Percentage
Abnormal tests	1	33.33%
AMI	1	33.33%
Diabetic Manifestations	1	33.33%
Total:	3	

CHAPTER 10

Retrospective Documentation Controls: Physician Queries

Retrospective Documentation Controls: Physician Queries

The best way to improve clinical documentation is through education and concurrent prompting while the subject patients are on the unit. However, every organization should also have a retrospective query process in place to ensure that if a documentation issue should slip through the cracks concurrently, it can still be salvaged retrospectively. This process, known as the physician query, must be implemented and consistent with the standards of local QIOs (quality improvement organizations). In this chapter, we will outline and interpret the regulations of the Centers for Medicare & Medicaid Services (CMS) that can help every organization implement an effective retrospective query process.

Background information on physician querying

Several official sources suggest when to query the physician. The American Health Information Management Association's Standards of Ethical Coding states, "Physicians should be consulted for clarification when they enter conflicting or ambiguous documentation in the chart" (Standard #6). The Department of Health and Human Services' Office of Inspector General recommends that coders communicate with physicians when documentation in the patient record is incomplete or unclear (*Compliance Guidance for Third Party Billing Companies*, 1999). The AHA *Coding Clinic* recommends that the physician be queried when documentation in the patient's record is "suggestive" of a condition but not clearly documented as such by the attending physician (Second Quarter 1998). Furthermore, *Coding Clinic* discusses the need for coders to identify "gaps in documentation where additional physician query may be necessary" (Second Quarter, 1998). With regard to abnormal laboratory findings, the National Center for Health Statistics' *Official Coding Guidelines for ICD-9-CM* states, "Abnormal findings (laboratory, x-ray, pathologic, and other diagnostic results) are not coded and reported unless the physician indicates their clinical significance. If the findings are outside the normal range and the

Chapter 10

physician has ordered other tests to evaluate the condition or prescribed treatment, it is appropriate to ask the physician whether the diagnosis should be added for accurate code assignment" (Guideline 3.5).

After assessing all official guidance regarding the physician query process, it appears that there is agreement that physicians should be queried when documentation is

- inconsistent or ambiguous
- unspecified or general in nature (when clinical clues may suggest more specific information)
- unclear
- incomplete
- supportive or suggestive of a certain clinical condition, but is not stated as such by the physician

Examples of each situation described above may provide further insight into the application of these official guidelines for when it is appropriate to query the physician.

In an example of inconsistent or ambiguous documentation, a physician sees a patient who has pneumonia. The doctor documents "viral pneumonia" in one progress note and "pneumococcal" in another. Of course, the coder needs to take all of the documentation into consideration. If the physician documented "viral" in an early progress note only once, followed by a stream of later progress notes (including the discharge progress note) where she or he documented "pneumoccocal," this probably does not indicate continuing inconsistency. Coders need to judge each case based upon their previous professional experience, education, and application of official coding guidelines.

Here's an example of both incomplete and general, or nonspecific, documentation, where the physician should be queried: A patient has pneumonia, and the physician has not specified what type. The labs show a positive culture and sensitivity for a particular organism.

The *Second Quarter 1998 Coding Clinic* states, "The coder should never assign a diagnosis based on a patient's signs and symptoms without confirmation by the physician. However, if a lab or radiology finding supports the selection of a more specific diagnosis than the physician has documented, then the physician should be queried to confirm that the more specific diagnosis may be used. In those cases where there is disagreement between the attending physician's final diagnosis and an examination report, the attending physician has the final word."

Don't conduct queries solely in situations with a potential to increase reimbursement. Doing so may create the appearance of a lack of concern for overall coding accuracy and of a focus on the bottom line only. In addition, conducting queries only when there is potential to increase reimbursement produces even further concerns.

Finally, healthcare providers should apply the physician query process to all types of records, not just inpatient records. While there is some level of cost-benefit analysis that each provider will undoubtedly use to determine the appropriate approach for querying physicians, strong consideration should be given to including the query process for all record types.

Each provider must have a written policy that clearly states when coders should query the physician. However, as noted above, you should handle each case based on its own documentation. In the end, application of the policy and the specific documentation in each record, coupled with the coder's experience, education, and application of the official coding guidelines, should result in appropriately timed queries.

Ten reasons to query physicians

In healthcare reimbursement, best practices dictate that all necessary documentation for coding should appear in the patient's record prior to discharge. With increasingly shortened lengths of stay and the need for physician education on the documentation process, obtaining necessary documentation prior to the patient's discharge is not always possible. If coders encounter incomplete, inconsistent, and unclear documentation, they'll need to communicate with the attending physician in order to clarify it. There are an infinite number of reasons for querying the physicians on your medical staff for documentation clarification; we've narrowed down the list to our top ten reasons:

1. Makes good business sense

In the reimbursement scheme, the physician is the "supplier" of documentation. The coder then takes that documentation and converts it into data elements that allow a bill to be created. In healthcare, as in any business, querying the physician (the supplier of your raw material) makes good business sense. In order for any business to be run effectively and efficiently, the components need to interact, or communicate. The physician query process does just that—it provides a forum whereby the supplier (the physician) and the converter of documentation (the coder) interact to ensure the highest-quality product possible.

2. Clarifies the difference between "book" versus "clinical" terminology

One of the longest-standing problems for physicians, even before the inpatient PPS was implemented, was the inconsistency between ICD-9-CM, or "book" language, and the natural clinical language used by physicians. This is a continuing concern, and it creates the potential for inaccuracy in coding if coders do not proactively query physicians for clarification.

3. Establishes which diagnoses to code when multiple physicians see the patient

Our official coding guidelines tell us that when multiple physicians are seeing the patient, the attending physician's documentation takes precedence over all others. Physicians, however, will argue this point and state that if they order a consult on a condition, then the consultant should be considered the expert, and his or her documentation should be relied upon. At times, coders may find that attending physicians have not documented conditions recorded by consultants. Coders may need to query attendings for further clarification on this issue.

4. Explains the significance of diagnostic tests

Official guidelines dictate that the coder may not code from diagnostic test results. Rather, the physician must document the significance of any test results. If the physician has neglected to document this information in the patient's record prior to discharge, but there is clinical evidence to support the fact that a particular condition may actually exist, then the coder should query the physician for verification.

5. Resolves documentation inconsistencies in different settings

A common scenario, especially for Medicare patients, is to be admitted initially to the emergency department (ED) and then transferred into the acute care setting. Often, coders may find information documented in the ED record that may not be present in the inpatient record. Without the ability to query the attending physician, this information may go uncoded, even though it may be a condition the physician treated, tested, or clinically evaluated.

6. Clarifies conflicting documentation from the same physician

Often, the same physician may provide information in the patient's record that conflicts with information she or he documented in another part of the patient's record. The coder will be stuck for a code without input from the physician in this circumstance.

7. Provides closure to coding a record with incomplete documentation

Patient records should be complete prior to coding, but often that is not the case. It's especially true with the discharge summary. Physicians need to understand the importance of including current information in the patient's record, and not just saving it all until the discharge summary. Many doctors will procrastinate, however. The physician who waits to tie up loose ends in the discharge summary creates problems for the coder and necessitates queries about documentation.

8. Provides clarification when physicians use "just plain old bad grammar"

Recently, our coding consulting staff came across the following statement by the attending physician in the discharge summary as his way of "clearly" documenting the patient's final diagnosis: "syncope secondary to ischemic colitis and SBO vs. intestinal abscess." This is a good example of poor grammar preventing good coding. Here, the coder can't tell whether the physician is stating that the syncope was due to all three conditions—in which case the principal diagnosis would be syncope, or if the syncope is due only to ischemic colitis—in which case the principal diagnosis would be ischemic colitis. Without asking the physician to clarify this statement, the record could not be coded accurately.

9. Educates the physician staff

Every provider wants to improve the reimbursement process in a "proactive" way. This means educating the physician. The physician query process can serve as ongoing training for your medical staff. After one physician has been queried three times about the same issue, he or she should begin to document the information correctly. A query isn't foolproof, but it is an effective mechanism for informing the physician.

10. Educates the coding staff

Coder interaction with physicians is one of the best ways to improve coders' knowledge of the clinical tasks behind coding and documentation. Generally, coders with this clinical knowledge are more likely to be better coders than their counterparts without that knowledge and training. The physician query process provides an excellent opportunity for coders to expand their knowledge base and become better coders. Figure 10.1 shows all ten reasons for querying physicians.

Figure 10.1 **Top Ten Reasons for Querying Physicians**

1. Makes good business sense
2. Clarifies the difference between "book" versus "clinical" terminology
3. Establishes which diagnoses should be coded when multiple physicians are seeing the patient
4. Explains the significance of diagnostic tests
5. Resolves documentation inconsistencies in different settings
6. Clarifies conflicting documentation from the same physician
7. Provides closure to coding a record with incomplete documentation
8. Provides clarification when physicians use "just plain old bad grammar"
9. Educates the physician staff
10. Educates the coding staff

Developing physician query policies and procedures

In order for any process to work well within an organization, it must embody the philosophy and culture of that organization. Without putting your own "stamp" on a policy or procedure, the possibility of its success is dismal. There are several steps that every organization needs to take to implement the physician query process effectively. We have outlined the bigger steps and the concepts that need to be addressed within each step.

Develop the format of your queries

You must determine, with some level of certainty, an acceptable query format in your organization. We have provided below some of the concepts that we encourage organizations to adopt. Again, remember that each decision must have your own organization's "stamp." We believe that these suggested formats are well within the (sometimes nebulous) guidelines provided to the healthcare industry, but they are not the only means available.

Develop a formal query process

You should acknowledge up front that the query process is a part of the record-keeping activities of your business. The query discusses clinical information about the patient and specifically identifies the patient. Under the CPRI definition of the patient's medical record, the physician query should be included as part of the patient's record. However, we acknowledge that at least one source would disagree with this conclusion, and until CMS or another official source determines otherwise, we would recommend keeping the query as part of the patient's clinical record. As a result, the following types of practices should be prohibited: scribbling a query to a physician on a "sticky" note or other piece of scratch paper or asking the physician verbally for confirmation of the query. We hope that the days of sloppy, unprofessional communications with physicians are history. The query is part of your business process, so it should include all the following necessary information on the document:

- Patient name
- Admission and discharge date
- Medical record number
- Physician name
- Coder name and signature
- Date of query
- Physician response
- Date of response
- Physician signature attesting to his or her response

Develop a specific format for queries

You should develop your own forms and formats for conducting the query process. The reason for this is twofold: First, the process will be much more reliable and efficient if your staff work from the same source document; second, physicians will become accustomed to the uniform format and may be able to work through the queries quicker. You may want to develop specific queries for certain diagnoses for which your coders make repeated queries. Repeating a query over and over should provide some additional training to physicians. Eventually, they will understand that if they do not want to be bothered with certain queries, they need to provide more specific documentation. However, even if coders query a physician on a new issue, they should use a format shared by your entire organization.

Prohibit "close-ended" queries except in specific situations

The idea of using an open-ended query whenever possible appeals to us. In light of the focus on federal False Claims Act investigations surrounding some coding practices, we believe it is important to ensure that coders are not using queries to lead physicians toward a certain response. An example of a close-ended query would be "Did the patient have gram negative pneumonia?" Asking the same question in an open-ended manner would be "Was the patient's pneumonia caused by a specific organism? If yes, please specify the organism." In this case, we would also support providing check boxes with the names of various organisms for the physician to choose from, as long as the choice included the terms "unspecified," "viral," or "unknown."

To avoid using leading questions, you can prohibit the use of close-ended queries except in specifically defined situations. The exceptions detailed in the *Coding Clinic* are a good basis for developing exceptions to the open-ended query process. It appears that only in the following circumstances is it appropriate to query for specific diagnoses (based upon *Coding Clinic* advice):

a. positive lab or radiology findings clinically supporting the diagnosis
b. medication is prescribed that supports the specific diagnosis

The *Coding Clinic* describes these instances when physicians could be queried regarding specific diseases. For example, *Coding Clinic Second Quarter 1998,* pages 4 and 5, states, "If a lab or radiology finding supports the selection of a more specific diagnosis than the physician has documented, then the physician should be queried to confirm that the more specific diagnoses may be used." And, *Coding Clinic First Quarter, 1993*, p. 24, states, "Coders should query the attending physician if, after reviewing the record, questions remain concerning prescribed medication that may indicate a specific condition." Finally, *Coding Clinic Second Quarter 1998* states, "Query the physician to confirm whether a [positive] culture finding identifies the causative organism [of the pneumonia]."

Develop other query guidelines specific to your organization

In addition to the issue of leading versus open-ended queries, you will need to develop other guidelines to apply to your organization's query process. These guidelines may be questions asked by your coders on a regular basis or may develop as you roll out the formal query process. They may also be guidelines that you develop in conjunction with your query team.

Write the process from start to finish in a policy and procedure

After you have determined the format of your queries and the rules that will apply to your process, you need to formalize this information in a policy and procedure. The policy and procedure should be written in a format that is easily understood by your coding and HIM staff. It should contain examples of good queries, sample query forms, and answers to common questions your coding staff or medical staff may ask regarding the query process.

Train your staff and the physicians on the query process

You cannot assume that coders will read, understand, or apply the information about the coding query process correctly simply because a management staff brought all of it together and translated it into a theoretically workable process. In fact, you should assume just the opposite. That is, unless you train and implement the process with your staff, it will not work, they will not understand it, and it will not be applied correctly in most situations. As you roll out the training process, you will also find that many questions are asked that will help you to continue to refine the process and make it even more workable. Remember that every policy and procedure should be dynamic, not a static, inflexible document that prevents coders from doing their jobs in the best way they can.

CHAPTER 11

Managing and Tracking Documentation

Managing and Tracking Documentation

Introduction

Every CDI program must be managed and tracked to ensure its ongoing effectiveness. The primary, but not sole, measure of a CDI program is the facility's CMI because it can change for reasons other than improved or poor documentation. However, once a CDI program is implemented, a change in CMI usually goes back to some other reason, such as a change in the medical-surgical mix. In this chapter, we will discuss the way you can use CMI to track and measure program effectiveness.

A review of the basics of CMI principles

CMI reflects the average measure of a weighted classification for grouping patient cases. In the inpatient world, CMI is the measure of the average DRG weight for cases paid under the inpatient PPS. Case mix index is an important measure for acute care hospitals because a hospital's CMI tells the world about the amount of resources used by the inpatient cases that the hospital treats. Many experts argue that CMI is an overall poor indicator of the severity of a patient's condition, but hospitals also use CMI internally for financial forecasting and planning. For these reasons, the accuracy and reliability of CMI is essential. Because CMI is derived almost entirely from ICD-9-CM coding, its reliability depends on the accuracy of the facility's coded data.

To arrive at a CMI, a facility needs to add the relative weights for the DRGs into which it assigns all inpatient cases. Then, it divides that number by the total number of inpatient cases. CMI can be calculated by year, quarter, or month. In addition, CMI can be calculated for all patients or just those reimbursed by Medicare.

CMS believes that CMI can change for one of three reasons:

1. Real CMI changes: These types of changes occur when the average resource use of Medicare patients changes. For example, the hospital may see an increase in medically necessary surgeries or it may have opened an open-heart unit, which would naturally increase CMI.

2. Coding effects changes: These result from changes in hospital coding of patient records. For example, a comprehensive training session may improve the skill of the coding staff, who are now more adept at identifying documentation in the patient record that needs coding.

3. Reclassification effect: These types of changes occur when the annual DRG reclassification and recalibration changes may not be budget neutral. It is doubtful that we will see any of these types of changes in the future because CMS has pledged to ensure that all DRG changes are budget neutral.

Identifying reasons for a CMI change

Events other than a change in coding or documentation practices can impact CMI; you need to identify those possible events. In addition, during CMI analysis, you need to determine whether you can attribute a change—especially a drop—in CMI to any of the following:

- A decrease in the ratio of surgical to medical cases
- The types of new physicians admitted to the medical staff could contribute to the CMI makeup
- Physicians seeing patients on an inpatient basis that could be seen as outpatients will decrease CMI (e.g. "non-acute" principal diagnoses)
- A facility with a greater proportion of cases in DRGs where CMS decreased relative weights in the current fiscal year

These are just some of the causes of a declining case mix. Often, a facility that is experiencing more than one of these issues simultaneously will see them clearly reflected in the case mix. To determine if these, or other, issues are playing a role in your CMI changes, you will need to perform a case mix analysis starting with the following basic steps:

1. Generate reports with inpatient data information for the current period in question as well as reports for at least two previous periods for comparative information.

2. Determine the proportion of surgical to medical DRGs.

3. Determine any other significant changes in DRG groupings. For example, an increase or decrease of more than 10% in cases assigned to a DRG for a particular period could result from new medical staff privileges.

Look at the table of relative weight changes in the most recent fiscal year and determine what proportion of your cases fall under those DRGs. If it exceeds 10%, a change in medical staffing may be the reason. Unfortunately, when CMS says they make relative weight changes "budget neutral," they mean the government's budget, not yours.

Analysis of a CMI

Capturing an average case mix for a patient type provides a benchmark that hospitals can use to gauge themselves. In addition, because CMI is in the public domain, providers can also benchmark against their peers throughout the nation. CMI is also closely tracked by many government entities including CMS and the OIG. Ultimately, the only mechanism for ensuring accurate and reliable CMI is to ensure accurate and reliable documentation and coding.

Each year, the government calculates CMI for all PPS cases for every healthcare provider in the country. The listing of CMI by hospital provider number is published publicly and can be found at *http://www.hcfa.gov/medicare/worksheet/CMI_LABE.TXT*. We have also included a copy of this listing in the appendix to this book. The listing allows you to identify the annual case mix for a hospital as long as you know the provider's ID number. If you don't have a listing of provider ID numbers, you can find this on the Internet at *http://www.hcfa.gov/stats/pufiles htm*. This site contains the listing of all Medicare provider ID numbers and the CMI for each provider for the previous year. In addition, we have provided a sample piece of the provider number listing in the Appendix to this book.

In general, CMI should be analyzed using the following parameters:

- Time period
- Peer comparison
- Internal CMI comparison

Time period

The CMI for more than one month of patient discharges should be aggregated for analysis. Depending on the size of your organization, you may need even more than a one-month period to ensure that the data is valid and representative. In smaller organizations, for example less than 150 beds, you may need to include at least one quarter's worth of data in your analysis. When a CDI program has been newly implemented, the tendency may be to analyze data every week or every day. The problem with this approach is that it focuses on too few cases for the numbers to be meaningful. We recommend that CMI be analyzed in the following increments to identify trends:

- Month by month
- Quarter by quarter
- Half year by half year
- Year by year

A sample report can be found in Figure 11.1.

Figure 11.1 **Documentation Improvement/CMI Maintenance**

- From month 3 through 6, CMI should stabilize as evidenced by the following:
    - Decrease in records needing to be audited for coding (<10%)
    - Decrease in records changed during documentation audit (<5%)
- Any change in monthly CMI >.005 should be directly traceable to a change in the supply of care, such as surgeons on leave, or a decrease in the number of joint replacements/CABGs

Figure 11.2

Documentation Improvement Tracking Mechanisms

Short-Term Tracking

- ➢ CMI pre- & post-coding audit
- ➢ Case manager physician query reports
- ➢ Monthly documentation audits

Long-Term Tracking

- ➢ CMI by physician/specialty
- ➢ Monthly CMI (all-payer and PPS-only)
- ➢ Decrease in records selected for monthly coding audits
- ➢ Decrease in records changed during monthly coding audits
- ➢ Decrease in records changed during monthly documentation audits

Peer comparison

CMI can also be analyzed using the data of other organizations. We referred above to publicly available data that your organization can use for comparative purposes. Other sources of data include

- state data warehouses
- American Hospital Association
- state hospital associations
- American Hospital Directory (AHD.com)

With peer comparison you can compare the following types of data elements:

- CMI
- CMI by medical versus surgical DRGs
- CMI by medical and surgical specialties

Internal CMI comparison

By using internal CMI comparison, you can identify possible reasons for change in CMI or you can begin to spot the potential documentation issues in certain areas. Examples of internal CMI comparison include the following:

- CMI by nursing unit
- CMI by physician group
- CMI by individual physician

Conclusion/Summary

It is important to compare your CMI both externally and internally. External comparison provides a "norm" for your organization to benchmark against. External norms can be used to drive your tactical and operational planning for future CMI management. From an internal perspective, it is also important to compare different CMI measures. One of the most important reasons for this relates to operational tracking. A comparison of internal measures (e.g. hospital CMI month by month or physician group by physician by physician group) can provide both motivation and performance feedback. Motivation is provided in the sense that the participants in the CDI program react to either an increase in CMI (by doing more of the same activity that caused the CMI to increase) or decrease (by improving performance to get the CMI back up to an acceptable level again). Finally, comparing and tracking CMI can provide ongoing feedback to the participants in a CDI program. For example, a low medical CMI in a given month may indicate to the clinical staff that the internal medicine physicians need more attention and interaction on the nursing units.

CHAPTER 12

Continuous Reassessment of Clinical Documentation

Continuous Reassessment of Clinical Documentation

Chapter 12

Introduction

Throughout this book we have reviewed the components necessary for a clinical documentation improvement program in the inpatient, acute care setting. We have provided suggestions for implementing CDI that focus on the physician, the nonphysician clinician, and the coding staff. In addition, we have provided sample "generic" tools to guide your CDI program development. We have also stressed the importance of developing a program that will function effectively in your organization. Every organization is unique, and it is important to recognize that when introducing such a new, wide-ranging program as clinical documentation improvement.

In the previous chapter, we addressed the use of CMI and other data analyses to manage and track your CDI program on an ongoing basis. Tracking through the use of effective data tools is an important component to the success of any program. The final phase of the tracking and management function is feedback to the individuals who are involved in breathing life into the program: the physicians, nonphysician clinicians, and coding staff. In this chapter we describe that assessment and feedback process.

Figure 12.1 lists the most important short-term and long-term action items for a CDI program. The last item under long-term actions, maintaining documentation and coding benchmarks at less than 5%, can be maintained in the long run only through continuous assessment and feedback to all parties involved in the process.

Figure 12.1

Short-term and long-term action items

Most important short-term CDI action items

- Supporting case management function
- Regular auditing of documentation on the units
- Regular auditing of coding
- Reinforcement with the medical staff

Most important long-term CDI action items

- Identifying and maintaining optimal and accurate CMI
- Extending documentation improvements to all care areas
- Maintaining documentation and coding audit benchmarks at greater than 5%

Physician assessment and feedback

Your medical staff is the key to success in documentation improvement. Without the cooperation and involvement of the physicians on your medical staff, the CDI program will not flourish. Most physicians seem to have a natural thirst for knowledge and learning. Because CDI is about continuous learning, this can be an appealing aspect of the program for physicians, especially if you present the program as one that affords the physicians the potential for continuous learning from a reimbursement and clinical perspective. One of the ways that you can position the program as a continuous learning experience is to let clinical and coding staff provide feedback, in a nonpunitive way, to individual physicians. In order for the feedback to be effective, it should contain the following types of information:

1. Feedback on professional fee documentation, coding and billing issues as well as hospital-related concerns.

2. Positive as well as negative findings. Physicians need to feel that what you are asking them to do is attainable. Showing them when they did the right thing will go a long way to obtaining their long-term commitment to the program.

3. Real-life examples of individual physicians' documentation, pointing out where specific documentation, if legitimately present in the patient, could have made a difference in both the physicians' billing as well as the hospital's.

4. One-on-one feedback with individual physicians. This is the most effective means of communicating. Sending physicians a "report" of findings is probably least effective.

5. A feedback format that is prioritized by physician. If, in your program development phase, you have identified the top-admitting physicians, those with the highest CMI, then you probably have a group of 10 to 15 physicians who impact most of your inpatient cases. Give these physicians the most amount of time and one-on-one education. The return will be well worth the investment you make.

Concurrent clinical reviewer assessment & feedback

While physicians are the key to success in CDI, your nonphysician clinicians are the backbone of the program. The clinicians are the individuals who ensure that information is delivered to physicians and that necessary responses (in the form of documentation) are provided. The clinicians involved in CDI implementation have most likely added CDI to their already long list of tasks. The CDI program manager will need to take this into consideration when designing the feedback process for the clinical reviewers. These folks need to see the positive outcome of their work. Most case managers or other CDI clinicians want to know what kind of a CMI impact their efforts have made. They want to know that the time they are spending is both worthwhile and recognized as such by somebody higher up in the organization. You can meet the needs of clinicians by giving them the feedback need.

1. Recognize the achievements of the CDI clinician team in an individual and an aggregate manner. One of the ways you can do this is at meetings of the entire

group by sharing success stories of individual clinicians. You may want to have them tell their own success stories, or you may want to pick out a few of the more significant stories where clinicians have been able to, for example, obtain additional documentation that impacted coding assignment from the most uncooperative physician on the staff.

2. Quantify the accomplishments of the individual clinicians as well as the clinicians as a group in terms of their impact on CDI. One of the ways to do this is by reviewing CMI by unit or by case manager, as discussed in the previous chapter.

3. When you have identified concerns on certain units, be ready with suggestions for improvement. But, in addition, obtain the feedback from the clinician about why certain conditions that are not optimal for CDI may exist on their unit. You and one or more of the clinicians may need to brainstorm to think of ways to overcome resistance from certain physicians or groups.

HIM coding staff assessment and feedback

The HIM coding staff is the catalyst in the CDI program, the folks on the front lines who are constantly in touch with current events that impact clinical documentation guidelines from a reimbursement perspective. Because these folks lead an important piece of the CDI effort, it is important to keep them in the loop at all times. They should attend meetings with the clinicians and physicians whenever possible, so that they feel like a part of the team. In addition to providing updated information for the CDI program and partaking in updating the CDI tools, the coders also play a role in performing retrospective CDI. Coders should be given feedback on their physician query process since this is an inherent part of the CDI program. Some of the concepts that you can work into the coder feedback process include the following:

1. Coders should share with each other some of their successes and challenges in querying physicians. This group of professionals has been dealing with physicians in this capacity for quite some time and therefore has considerable experience in the process. Coders should be able to share any changes that have occurred in the process since physicians are being queried not only on the back end of the process now, but also at the point of service.

2. Review with the coding staff the actual format of the queries themselves. This review should be performed for many reasons, primarily to ensure compliant queries, understandable queries, and queries about whether sufficient clinical evidence existed in the record to support the queries in the first place.

Conclusion

As you go forward with your CDI program, keep in mind that the inpatient, acute care setting is only one place to implement CDI. Clinical documentation of a patient's care is of paramount importance regardless of the type or location of the care provided. The illustrations in Figure 12.2 depict the full extent of documentation improvement.

Figure 12.2 The Reach of Documentation Improvement

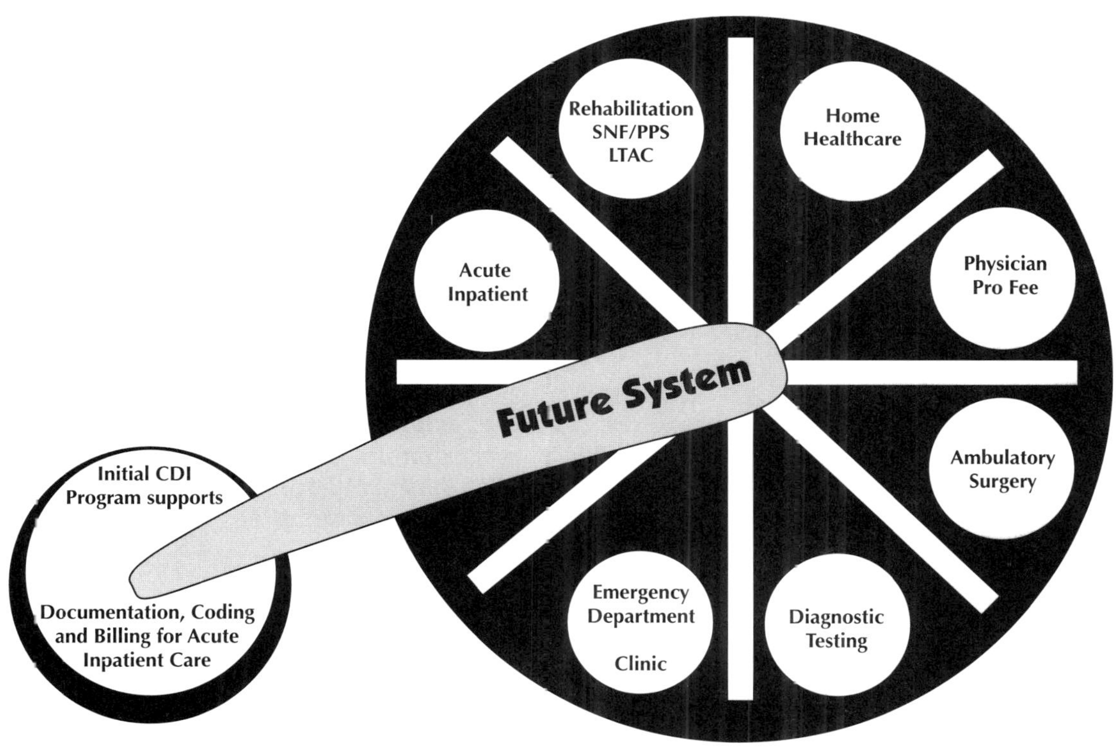

APPENDIX

Appendix

Appendix

Appendix 1

Conditions of Participation

§ 482.23 Condition of participation: Nursing services.

The hospital must have an organized nursing service that provides 24-hour nursing services. The nursing services must be furnished or supervised by a registered nurse.

(a) *Standard: Organization.* The hospital must have a well-organized service with a plan of administrative authority and delineation of responsibilities for patient care. The director of the nursing service must be a licensed registered nurse. He or she is responsible for the operation of the service, including determining the types and numbers of nursing personnel and staff necessary to provide nursing care for all areas of the hospital.

(b) *Standard: Staffing and delivery of care.* The nursing service must have adequate numbers of licensed registered nurses, licensed practical (vocational) nurses, and other personnel to provide nursing care to all patients as needed. There must be supervisory and staff personnel for each department or nursing unit to ensure, when needed, the immediate availability of a registered nurse for bedside care of any patient.

(1) The hospital must provide 24-hour nursing services furnished or supervised by a registered nurse, and have a licensed practical nurse or registered nurse on duty at all times, except for rural hospitals that have in effect a 24-hour nursing waiver granted under § 405.1910(c) of this chapter.

(2) The nursing service must have a procedure to ensure that hospital nursing personnel for whom licensure is required have valid and current licensure.

(3) A registered nurse must supervise and evaluate the nursing care for each patient.

(4) The hospital must ensure that the nursing staff develops, and keeps current, a nursing care plan for each patient.

(5) A registered nurse must assign the nursing care of each patient to other nursing personnel in accordance with the patient's needs and the specialized qualifications and competence of the nursing staff available.

(6) Non-employee licensed nurses who are working in the hospital must adhere to the policies and procedures of the hospital. The director of nursing service must provide for the adequate supervision and evaluation of the clinical activities of non-employee nursing personnel which occur within the responsibility of the nursing service.

(c) *Standard: Preparation and administration of drugs.* Drugs and biologicals must be prepared and administered in accordance with Federal and State laws, the orders of the practitioner or practitioners responsible for the patient's care as specified under § 482.12(c), and accepted standards of practice.

(1) All drugs and biologicals must be administered by, or under supervision of, nursing or other personnel in accordance with Federal and State laws and regulations, including applicable licensing requirements, and in accordance with the approved medical staff policies and procedures.

(2) All orders for drugs and biologicals must be in writing and signed by the practitioner or practitioners responsible for the care of the patient as specified under § 482.12(c). When telephone or oral orders must be used, they must be—

(i) Accepted only by personnel that are authorized to do so by the medical staff policies and procedures, consistent with Federal and State law;

(ii) Signed or initialed by the prescribing practitioner as soon as possible; and

(iii) Used infrequently.

(3) Blood transfusions and intravenous medications must be administered in accordance with State law and approved medical staff policies and procedures. If blood transfusions and intravenous medications are administered by personnel other than doctors of medicine or osteopathy, the personnel must have special training for this duty.

(4) There must be a hospital procedure for reporting transfusion reactions, adverse drug reactions, and errors in administration of drugs.

§ 482.24 Condition of participation: Medical record services.

The hospital must have a medical record service that has administrative responsibility for medical records. A

Appendix 1

Conditions of Participation (cont.)

medical record must be maintained for every individual evaluated or treated in the hospital.

(a) *Standard: Organization and staffing.* The organization of the medical record service must be appropriate to the scope and complexity of the services performed. The hospital must employ adequate personnel to ensure prompt completion, filing, and retrieval of records.

(b) *Standard: Form and retention of record.* The hospital must maintain a medical record for each inpatient and outpatient. Medical records must be accurately written, promptly completed, properly filed and retained, and accessible. The hospital must use a system of author identification and record maintenance that ensures the integrity of the authentification and protects the security of all record entries.

(1) Medical records must be retained in their original or legally reproduced form for a period of at least 5 years.

(2) The hospital must have a system of coding and indexing medical records. The system must allow for timely retrieval by diagnosis and procedure, in order to support medical care evaluation studies.

(3) The hospital must have a procedure for ensuring the confidentiality of patient records. In-formation from or copies of records may be released only to authorized individuals, and the hospital must ensure that unauthorized individuals cannot gain access to or alter patient records. Original medical records must be released by the hospital only in accordance with Federal or State laws, court orders, or subpoenas.

(c) *Standard: Content of record.* The medical record must contain information to justify admission and continued hospitalization, support the diagnosis, and describe the patient's progress and response to medications and services.

(1) All entries must be legible and complete, and must be authenticated and dated promptly by the person (identified by name and discipline) who is responsible for ordering, providing, or evaluating the service furnished.

(i) The author of each entry must be identifed and must authenticate his or her entry.

(ii) Authentication may include signatures, written initials or computer entry.

(2) All records must document the following, as appropriate:

(i) Evidence of a physical examination, including a health history, performed no more than 7 days prior to admission or within 48 hours after admission.

(ii) Admitting diagnosis.

(iii) Results of all consultative evaluations of the patient and appropriate findings by clinical and other staff involved in the care of the patient.

(iv) Documentation of complications, hospital acquired infections, and unfavorable reactions to drugs and anesthesia.

(v) Properly executed informed consent forms for procedures and treatments specified by the medical staff, or by Federal or State law if applicable, to require written patient consent.

(vi) All practitioners' orders, nursing notes, reports of treatment, medication records, radiology, and laboratory reports, and vital signs and other information necessary to monitor the patient's condition.

(vii) Discharge summary with outcome of hospitalization, disposition of case, and provisions for follow-up care.

(viii) Final diagnosis with completion of medical records within 30 days following discharge.

§ 482.25 Condition of participation: Pharmaceutical services.

The hospital must have pharmaceutical services that meet the needs of the patients. The institution must have a pharmacy directed by a registered pharmacist or a drug storage area under competent supervision. The medical staff is responsible for developing policies and procedures that minimize drug errors. This function may be delegated to the hospital's organized pharmaceutical service.

(a) *Standard: Pharmacy management and administration.* The pharmacy or drug storage area must be administered in accordance with accepted professional principles.

(1) A full-time, part-time, or consulting pharmacist must be responsible

Appendix 2

DRG Weights

DRG WEIGHTS

DRG	DRG Name	Weight
001	CRANIOTOMY AGE >17 EXCEPT FOR TRAUMA	3.2713
002	CRANIOTOMY FOR TRAUMA AGE >17	3.3874
003	CRANIOTOMY AGE 0-17	1.9594
004	SPINAL PROCEDURES	2.4148
005	EXTRACRANIAL VASCULAR PROCEDURES	1.3628
006	CARPAL TUNNEL RELEASE	0.7230
007	PERIPH & CRANIAL NERVE & OTHER NERV SYST PROC W CC	2.6285
008	PERIPH & CRANIAL NERVE & OTHER NERV SYST PROC W/O CC	1.3953
009	SPINAL DISORDERS & INJURIES	1.3350
010	NERVOUS SYSTEM NEOPLASMS W CC	1.2690
011	NERVOUS SYSTEM NEOPLASMS W/O CC	0.8471
012	DEGENERATIVE NERVOUS SYSTEM DISORDERS	0.9020
013	MULTIPLE SCLEROSIS & CEREBELLAR ATAXIA	0.8129
014	SPECIFIC CEREBROVASCULAR DISORDERS EXCEPT TIA	1.1655
015	TRANSIENT ISCHEMIC ATTACK & PRECEREBRAL OCCLUSIONS	0.7349
016	NONSPECIFIC CEREBROVASCULAR DISORDERS W CC	1.1867
017	NONSPECIFIC CEREBROVASCULAR DISORDERS W/O CC	0.6689
018	CRANIAL & PERIPHERAL NERVE DISORDERS W CC	0.9744
019	CRANIAL & PERIPHERAL NERVE DISORDERS W/O CC	0.6756
020	NERVOUS SYSTEM INFECTION EXCEPT VIRAL MENINGITIS	2.7764
021	VIRAL MENINGITIS	1.4573
022	HYPERTENSIVE ENCEPHALOPATHY	1.0037
023	NONTRAUMATIC STUPOR & COMA	0.8069
024	SEIZURE & HEADACHE AGE >17 W CC	1.0172
025	SEIZURE & HEADACHE AGE >17 W/O CC	0.5947
026	SEIZURE & HEADACHE AGE 0-17	0.5981
027	TRAUMATIC STUPOR & COMA, COMA >1 HR	1.3514
028	TRAUMATIC STUPOR & COMA, COMA <1 HR AGE >17 W CC	1.3609
029	TRAUMATIC STUPOR & COMA, COMA <1 HR AGE >17 W/O CC	0.6956

Appendix 2

DRG Weights (cont.)

DRG	DRG Name	Weight
030	TRAUMATIC STUPOR & COMA, COMA <1 HR AGE 0-17	0.3314
031	CONCUSSION AGE >17 W CC	0.9165
032	CONCUSSION AGE >17 W/O CC	0.5230
033	CONCUSSION AGE 0-17	0.2082
034	OTHER DISORDERS OF NERVOUS SYSTEM W CC	1.0074
035	OTHER DISORDERS OF NERVOUS SYSTEM W/O CC	0.5885
036	RETINAL PROCEDURES	0.6615
037	ORBITAL PROCEDURES	1.1300
038	PRIMARY IRIS PROCEDURES	0.4751
039	LENS PROCEDURES WITH OR WITHOUT VITRECTOMY	0.5986
040	EXTRAOCULAR PROCEDURES EXCEPT ORBIT AGE >17	0.8264
041	EXTRAOCULAR PROCEDURES EXCEPT ORBIT AGE 0-17	0.3374
042	INTRAOCULAR PROCEDURES EXCEPT RETINA, IRIS & LENS	0.6302
043	HYPHEMA	0.4578
044	ACUTE MAJOR EYE INFECTIONS	0.6554
045	NEUROLOGICAL EYE DISORDERS	0.6760
046	OTHER DISORDERS OF THE EYE AGE >17 W CC	0.7962
047	OTHER DISORDERS OF THE EYE AGE >17 W/O CC	0.5043
048	OTHER DISORDERS OF THE EYE AGE 0-17	0.2972
049	MAJOR HEAD & NECK PROCEDURES	1.7649
050	SIALOADENECTOMY	0.8158
051	SALIVARY GLAND PROCEDURES EXCEPT SIALOADENECTOMY	0.7895
052	CLEFT LIP & PALATE REPAIR	0.7590
053	SINUS & MASTOID PROCEDURES AGE >17	1.1773
054	SINUS & MASTOID PROCEDURES AGE 0-17	0.4817
055	MISCELLANEOUS EAR, NOSE, MOUTH & THROAT PROCEDURES	0.8483
056	RHINOPLASTY	0.8787
057	T&A PROC, EXCEPT TONSILLECTOMY &/OR ADENOIDECTOMY ONLY, AGE >17	1.2004
058	T&A PROC, EXCEPT TONSILLECTOMY &/OR ADENOIDECTOMY ONLY, AGE 0-17	0.2735

Appendix 2

DRG Weights (cont.)

DRG	DRG Name	Weight
059	TONSILLECTOMY &/OR ADENOIDECTOMY ONLY, AGE >17	0.8276
060	TONSILLECTOMY &/OR ADENOIDECTOMY ONLY, AGE 0-17	0.2083
061	MYRINGOTOMY W TUBE INSERTION AGE >17	1.3541
062	MYRINGOTOMY W TUBE INSERTION AGE 0-17	0.2950
063	OTHER EAR, NOSE, MOUTH & THROAT O.R. PROCEDURES	1.3718
064	EAR, NOSE, MOUTH & THROAT MALIGNANCY	1.2319
065	DYSEQUILIBRIUM	0.5326
066	EPISTAXIS	0.5536
067	EPIGLOTTITIS	0.7514
068	OTITIS MEDIA & URI AGE >17 W CC	0.6665
069	OTITIS MEDIA & URI AGE >17 W/O CC	0.4948
070	OTITIS MEDIA & URI AGE 0-17	0.4575
071	LARYNGOTRACHEITIS	0.6685
072	NASAL TRAUMA & DEFORMITY	0.6699
073	OTHER EAR, NOSE, MOUTH & THROAT DIAGNOSES AGE >17	0.7993
074	OTHER EAR, NOSE, MOUTH & THROAT DIAGNOSES AGE 0-17	0.3352
075	MAJOR CHEST PROCEDURES	3.2096
076	OTHER RESP SYSTEM O.R. PROCEDURES W CC	3.0129
077	OTHER RESP SYSTEM O.R. PROCEDURES W/O CC	1.2416
078	PULMONARY EMBOLISM	1.3295
079	RESPIRATORY INFECTIONS & INFLAMMATIONS AGE >17 W CC	1.7094
080	RESPIRATORY INFECTIONS & INFLAMMATIONS AGE >17 W/O CC	0.9215
081	RESPIRATORY INFECTIONS & INFLAMMATIONS AGE 0-17	1.5177
082	RESPIRATORY NEOPLASMS	1.4316
083	MAJOR CHEST TRAUMA W CC	0.9803
084	MAJOR CHEST TRAUMA W/O CC	0.5454
085	PLEURAL EFFUSION W CC	1.2483
086	PLEURAL EFFUSION W/O CC	0.6769
087	PULMONARY EDEMA & RESPIRATORY FAILURE	1.4282
088	CHRONIC OBSTRUCTIVE PULMONARY DISEASE	0.9127

Appendix 2

DRG Weights (cont.)

DRG	DRG Name	Weight
089	SIMPLE PNEUMONIA & PLEURISY AGE >17 W CC	1.0601
090	SIMPLE PNEUMONIA & PLEURISY AGE >17 W/O CC	0.6344
091	SIMPLE PNEUMONIA & PLEURISY AGE 0-17	0.7937
092	INTERSTITIAL LUNG DISEASE W CC	1.2296
093	INTERSTITIAL LUNG DISEASE W/O CC	0.7443
094	PNEUMOTHORAX W CC	1.2024
095	PNEUMOTHORAX W/O CC	0.5817
096	BRONCHITIS & ASTHMA AGE >17 W CC	0.7604
097	BRONCHITIS & ASTHMA AGE >17 W/O CC	0.5636
098	BRONCHITIS & ASTHMA AGE 0-17	0.7496
099	RESPIRATORY SIGNS & SYMPTOMS W CC	0.6964
100	RESPIRATORY SIGNS & SYMPTOMS W/O CC	0.5186
101	OTHER RESPIRATORY SYSTEM DIAGNOSES W CC	0.8604
102	OTHER RESPIRATORY SYSTEM DIAGNOSES W/O CC	0.5207
103	HEART TRANSPLANT	20.2413
104	CARDIAC VALVE & OTH MAJOR CARDIOTHORACIC PROC W CARD CATH	7.8411
105	CARDIAC VALVE & OTH MAJOR CARDIOTHORACIC PROC W/O CARD CATH	5.6796
106	CORONARY BYPASS W PTCA	7.4396
107	CORONARY BYPASS W CARDIAC CATH	5.3125
108	OTHER CARDIOTHORACIC PROCEDURES	5.5325
109	CORONARY BYPASS W/O PTCA OR CARDIAC CATH	3.9017
110	MAJOR CARDIOVASCULAR PROCEDURES W CC	4.1576
111	MAJOR CARDIOVASCULAR PROCEDURES W/O CC	2.2865
112	NO LONGER VALID	0.0000
113	AMPUTATION FOR CIRC SYSTEM DISORDERS EXCEPT UPPER LIMB & TOE	2.6714
114	UPPER LIMB & TOE AMPUTATION FOR CIRC SYSTEM DISORDERS	1.6809
115	PRM CARD PACEM IMPL W AMI,HRT FAIL OR SHK,OR AICD LEAD OR GN	3.3822
116	OTHER PERMANENT CARDIAC PACEMAKER IMPLANT	2.2648

Appendix 2

DRG Weights (cont.)

DRG	DRG Name	Weight
117	CARDIAC PACEMAKER REVISION EXCEPT DEVICE REPLACEMENT	1.3351
118	CARDIAC PACEMAKER DEVICE REPLACEMENT	1.4339
119	VEIN LIGATION & STRIPPING	1.3578
120	OTHER CIRCULATORY SYSTEM O.R. PROCEDURES	2.3552
121	CIRCULATORY DISORDERS W AMI & MAJOR COMP, DISCHARGED ALIVE	1.5787
122	CIRCULATORY DISORDERS W AMI W/O MAJOR COMP, DISCHARGED ALIVE	1.0241
123	CIRCULATORY DISORDERS W AMI, EXPIRED	1.5883
124	CIRCULATORY DISORDERS EXCEPT AMI, W CARD CATH & COMPLEX DIAG	1.4072
125	CIRCULATORY DISORDERS EXCEPT AMI, W CARD CATH W/O COMPLEX DIAG	1.0406
126	ACUTE & SUBACUTE ENDOCARDITIS	2.6836
127	HEART FAILURE & SHOCK	1.0103
128	DEEP VEIN THROMBOPHLEBITIS	0.7320
129	CARDIAC ARREST, UNEXPLAINED	1.0209
130	PERIPHERAL VASCULAR DISORDERS W CC	0.9379
131	PERIPHERAL VASCULAR DISORDERS W/O CC	0.5725
132	ATHEROSCLEROSIS W CC	0.6473
133	ATHEROSCLEROSIS W/O CC	0.5558
134	HYPERTENSION	0.5814
135	CARDIAC CONGENITAL & VALVULAR DISORDERS AGE >17 W CC	0.9128
136	CARDIAC CONGENITAL & VALVULAR DISORDERS AGE >17 W/O CC	0.5643
137	CARDIAC CONGENITAL & VALVULAR DISORDERS AGE 0-17	0.8177
138	CARDIAC ARRHYTHMIA & CONDUCTION DISORDERS W CC	0.8222
139	CARDIAC ARRHYTHMIA & CONDUCTION DISORDERS W/O CC	0.4961
140	ANGINA PECTORIS	0.5335
141	SYNCOPE & COLLAPSE W CC	0.7241
142	SYNCOPE & COLLAPSE W/O CC	0.5395
143	CHEST PAIN	0.5191
144	OTHER CIRCULATORY SYSTEM DIAGNOSES W CC	1.2015

Appendix 2

DRG Weights (cont.)

DRG	DRG Name	Weight
145	OTHER CIRCULATORY SYSTEM DIAGNOSES W/O CC	0.5899
146	RECTAL RESECTION W CC	2.7764
147	RECTAL RESECTION W/O CC	1.5993
148	MAJOR SMALL & LARGE BOWEL PROCEDURES W CC	3.5332
149	MAJOR SMALL & LARGE BOWEL PROCEDURES W/O CC	1.5063
150	PERITONEAL ADHESIOLYSIS W CC	2.9483
151	PERITONEAL ADHESIOLYSIS W/O CC	1.3451
152	MINOR SMALL & LARGE BOWEL PROCEDURES W CC	1.9477
153	MINOR SMALL & LARGE BOWEL PROCEDURES W/O CC	1.1642
154	STOMACH, ESOPHAGEAL & DUODENAL PROCEDURES AGE >17 W CC	4.3519
155	STOMACH, ESOPHAGEAL & DUODENAL PROCEDURES AGE >17 W/O CC	1.3273
156	STOMACH, ESOPHAGEAL & DUODENAL PROCEDURES AGE 0-17	0.8421
157	ANAL & STOMAL PROCEDURES W CC	1.2599
158	ANAL & STOMAL PROCEDURES W/O CC	0.6209
159	HERNIA PROCEDURES EXCEPT INGUINAL & FEMORAL AGE >17 W CC	1.3618
160	HERNIA PROCEDURES EXCEPT INGUINAL & FEMORAL AGE >17 W/O CC	0.7655
161	INGUINAL & FEMORAL HERNIA PROCEDURES AGE >17 W CC	1.1375
162	INGUINAL & FEMORAL HERNIA PROCEDURES AGE >17 W/O CC	0.6121
163	HERNIA PROCEDURES AGE 0-17	0.6909
164	APPENDECTOMY W COMPLICATED PRINCIPAL DIAG W CC	2.3960
165	APPENDECTOMY W COMPLICATED PRINCIPAL DIAG W/O CC	1.2904
166	APPENDECTOMY W/O COMPLICATED PRINCIPAL DIAG W CC	1.4934
167	APPENDECTOMY W/O COMPLICATED PRINCIPAL DIAG W/O CC	0.8753
168	MOUTH PROCEDURES W CC	1.2982
169	MOUTH PROCEDURES W/O CC	0.6964
170	OTHER DIGESTIVE SYSTEM O.R. PROCEDURES W CC	3.0540
171	OTHER DIGESTIVE SYSTEM O.R. PROCEDURES W/O CC	1.1716
172	DIGESTIVE MALIGNANCY W CC	1.3985

Appendix 2

DRG Weights (cont.)

DRG	DRG Name	Weight
173	DIGESTIVE MALIGNANCY W/O CC	0.6933
174	G.I. HEMORRHAGE W CC	0.9896
175	G.I. HEMORRHAGE W/O CC	0.5419
176	COMPLICATED PEPTIC ULCER	1.0888
177	UNCOMPLICATED PEPTIC ULCER W CC	0.8910
178	UNCOMPLICATED PEPTIC ULCER W/O CC	0.6408
179	INFLAMMATORY BOWEL DISEASE	1.0868
180	G.I. OBSTRUCTION W CC	0.9565
181	G.I. OBSTRUCTION W/O CC	0.5237
182	ESOPHAGITIS, GASTROENT & MISC DIGEST DISORDERS AGE >17 W CC	0.7940
183	ESOPHAGITIS, GASTROENT & MISC DIGEST DISORDERS AGE >17 W/O CC	0.5568
184	ESOPHAGITIS, GASTROENT & MISC DIGEST DISORDERS AGE 0-17	0.4141
185	DENTAL & ORAL DIS EXCEPT EXTRACTIONS & RESTORATIONS, AGE >17	0.8660
186	DENTAL & ORAL DIS EXCEPT EXTRACTIONS & RESTORATIONS, AGE 0-17	0.3210
187	DENTAL EXTRACTIONS & RESTORATIONS	0.7868
188	OTHER DIGESTIVE SYSTEM DIAGNOSES AGE >17 W CC	1.1250
189	OTHER DIGESTIVE SYSTEM DIAGNOSES AGE >17 W/O CC	0.5776
190	OTHER DIGESTIVE SYSTEM DIAGNOSES AGE 0-17	1.1897
191	PANCREAS, LIVER & SHUNT PROCEDURES W CC	4.6199
192	PANCREAS, LIVER & SHUNT PROCEDURES W/O CC	1.8255
193	BILIARY TRACT PROC EXCEPT ONLY CHOLECYST W OR W/O C.D.E. W CC	3.5085
194	BILIARY TRACT PROC EXCEPT ONLY CHOLECYST W OR W/O C.D.E. W/O CC	1.7294
195	CHOLECYSTECTOMY W C.D.E. W CC	3.0863
196	CHOLECYSTECTOMY W C.D.E. W/O CC	1.6111
197	CHOLECYSTECTOMY EXCEPT BY LAPAROSCOPE W/O C.D.E. W CC	2.5748
198	CHOLECYSTECTOMY EXCEPT BY LAPAROSCOPE W/O C.D.E. W/O CC	1.2062
199	HEPATOBILIARY DIAGNOSTIC PROCEDURE FOR MALIGNANCY	2.5070

Appendix 2

DRG Weights (cont.)

DRG	DRG Name	Weight
200	HEPATOBILIARY DIAGNOSTIC PROCEDURE FOR NON-MALIGNANCY	3.1811
201	OTHER HEPATOBILIARY OR PANCREAS O.R. PROCEDURES	3.7986
202	CIRRHOSIS & ALCOHOLIC HEPATITIS	1.3291
203	MALIGNANCY OF HEPATOBILIARY SYSTEM OR PANCREAS	1.3627
204	DISORDERS OF PANCREAS EXCEPT MALIGNANCY	1.2047
205	DISORDERS OF LIVER EXCEPT MALIG,CIRR,ALC HEPA W CC	1.2207
206	DISORDERS OF LIVER EXCEPT MALIG,CIRR,ALC HEPA W/O CC	0.7302
207	DISORDERS OF THE BILIARY TRACT W CC	1.1120
208	DISORDERS OF THE BILIARY TRACT W/O CC	0.6380
209	MAJOR JOINT & LIMB REATTACHMENT PROCEDURES OF LOWER EXTREMITY	1.9917
210	HIP & FEMUR PROCEDURES EXCEPT MAJOR JOINT AGE >17 W CC	1.7503
211	HIP & FEMUR PROCEDURES EXCEPT MAJOR JOINT AGE >17 W/O CC	1.2236
212	HIP & FEMUR PROCEDURES EXCEPT MAJOR JOINT AGE 0-17	0.8457
213	AMPUTATION FOR MUSCULOSKELETAL SYSTEM & CONN TISSUE DISORDERS	1.9437
214	NO LONGER VALID	0.0000
215	NO LONGER VALID	0.0000
216	BIOPSIES OF MUSCULOSKELETAL SYSTEM & CONNECTIVE TISSUE	2.3172
217	WND DEBRID & SKN GRFT EXCEPT HAND,FOR MUSCSKELET & CONN TISS DIS	3.2005
218	LOWER EXTREM & HUMER PROC EXCEPT HIP,FOOT,FEMUR AGE >17 W CC	1.5499
219	LOWER EXTREM & HUMER PROC EXCEPT HIP,FOOT,FEMUR AGE >17 W/O CC	0.9950
220	LOWER EXTREM & HUMER PROC EXCEPT HIP,FOOT,FEMUR AGE 0-17	0.5834
221	NO LONGER VALID	0.0000
222	NO LONGER VALID	0.0000
223	MAJOR SHOULDER/ELBOW PROC, OR OTHER UPPER EXTREMITY PROC W CC	0.9723
224	SHOULDER,ELBOW OR FOREARM PROC,EXC MAJOR JOINT PROC, W/O CC	0.7697

Appendix 2

DRG Weights (cont.)

DRG	DRG Name	Weight
225	FOOT PROCEDURES	1.1164
226	SOFT TISSUE PROCEDURES W CC	1.5902
227	SOFT TISSUE PROCEDURES W/O CC	0.7922
228	MAJOR THUMB OR JOINT PROC,OR OTH HAND OR WRIST PROC W CC	1.0906
229	HAND OR WRIST PROC, EXCEPT MAJOR JOINT PROC, W/O CC	0.7142
230	LOCAL EXCISION & REMOVAL OF INT FIX DEVICES OF HIP & FEMUR	1.3598
231	LOCAL EXCISION & REMOVAL OF INT FIX DEVICES EXCEPT HIP & FEMUR	1.4340
232	ARTHROSCOPY	0.9532
233	OTHER MUSCULOSKELET SYS & CONN TISS O.R. PROC W CC	2.0945
234	OTHER MUSCULOSKELET SYS & CONN TISS O.R. PROC W/O CC	1.2097
235	FRACTURES OF FEMUR	0.7632
236	FRACTURES OF HIP & PELVIS	0.6889
237	SPRAINS, STRAINS, & DISLOCATIONS OF HIP, PELVIS & THIGH	0.5325
238	OSTEOMYELITIS	1.4154
239	PATHOLOGICAL FRACTURES & MUSCULOSKELETAL & CONN TISS MALIGNANCY	1.0032
240	CONNECTIVE TISSUE DISORDERS W CC	1.3692
241	CONNECTIVE TISSUE DISORDERS W/O CC	0.6315
242	SEPTIC ARTHRITIS	1.0953
243	MEDICAL BACK PROBLEMS	0.7304
244	BONE DISEASES & SPECIFIC ARTHROPATHIES W CC	0.7152
245	BONE DISEASES & SPECIFIC ARTHROPATHIES W/O CC	0.4665
246	NON-SPECIFIC ARTHROPATHIES	0.5717
247	SIGNS & SYMPTOMS OF MUSCULOSKELETAL SYSTEM & CONN TISSUE	0.5587
248	TENDONITIS, MYOSITIS & BURSITIS	0.8160
249	AFTERCARE, MUSCULOSKELETAL SYSTEM & CONNECTIVE TISSUE	0.6784
250	FX, SPRN, STRN & DISL OF FOREARM, HAND, FOOT AGE >17 W CC	0.6809
251	FX, SPRN, STRN & DISL OF FOREARM, HAND, FOOT AGE >17 W/O CC	0.4582
252	FX, SPRN, STRN & DISL OF FOREARM, HAND, FOOT AGE 0-17	0.2533

Appendix 2

DRG Weights (cont.)

DRG	DRG Name	Weight
253	FX, SPRN, STRN & DISL OF UPARM,LOWLEG EX FOOT AGE >17 W CC	0.7397
254	FX, SPRN, STRN & DISL OF UPARM,LOWLEG EX FOOT AGE >17 W/O CC	0.4294
255	FX, SPRN, STRN & DISL OF UPARM,LOWLEG EX FOOT AGE 0-17	0.2951
256	OTHER MUSCULOSKELETAL SYSTEM & CONNECTIVE TISSUE DIAGNOSES	0.8152
257	TOTAL MASTECTOMY FOR MALIGNANCY W CC	0.8783
258	TOTAL MASTECTOMY FOR MALIGNANCY W/O CC	0.6954
259	SUBTOTAL MASTECTOMY FOR MALIGNANCY W CC	0.8763
260	SUBTOTAL MASTECTOMY FOR MALIGNANCY W/O CC	0.6435
261	BREAST PROC FOR NON-MALIGNANCY EXCEPT BIOPSY & LOCAL EXCISION	0.9240
262	BREAST BIOPSY & LOCAL EXCISION FOR NON-MALIGNANCY	0.8487
263	SKIN GRAFT &/OR DEBRID FOR SKN ULCER OR CELLULITIS W CC	2.0570
264	SKIN GRAFT &/OR DEBRID FOR SKN ULCER OR CELLULITIS W/O CC	1.1079
265	SKIN GRAFT &/OR DEBRID EXCEPT FOR SKIN ULCER OR CELLULITIS W CC	1.6795
266	SKIN GRAFT &/OR DEBRID EXCEPT FOR SKIN ULCER OR CELLULITIS W/O CC	0.8414
267	PERIANAL & PILONIDAL PROCEDURES	0.9406
268	SKIN, SUBCUTANEOUS TISSUE & BREAST PLASTIC PROCEDURES	1.2368
269	OTHER SKIN, SUBCUT TISS & BREAST PROC W CC	1.7731
270	OTHER SKIN, SUBCUT TISS & BREAST PROC W/O CC	0.7806
271	SKIN ULCERS	1.0365
272	MAJOR SKIN DISORDERS W CC	1.0248
273	MAJOR SKIN DISORDERS W/O CC	0.5638
274	MALIGNANT BREAST DISORDERS W CC	1.1927
275	MALIGNANT BREAST DISORDERS W/O CC	0.6647
276	NON-MALIGANT BREAST DISORDERS	0.7033
277	CELLULITIS AGE >17 W CC	0.8534
278	CELLULITIS AGE >17 W/O CC	0.5487
279	CELLULITIS AGE 0-17	0.6632

Appendix 2

DRG Weights (cont.)

DRG	DRG Name	Weight
280	TRAUMA TO THE SKIN, SUBCUT TISS & BREAST AGE >17 W CC	0.6941
281	TRAUMA TO THE SKIN, SUBCUT TISS & BREAST AGE >17 W/O CC	0.4593
282	TRAUMA TO THE SKIN, SUBCUT TISS & BREAST AGE 0-17	0.2565
283	MINOR SKIN DISORDERS W CC	0.7152
284	MINOR SKIN DISORDERS W/O CC	0.4204
285	AMPUTAT OF LOWER LIMB FOR ENDOCRINE,NUTRIT,& METABOL DISORDERS	2.1297
286	ADRENAL & PITUITARY PROCEDURES	2.2343
287	SKIN GRAFTS & WOUND DEBRID FOR ENDOC, NUTRIT & METAB DISORDERS	1.9569
288	O.R. PROCEDURES FOR OBESITY	2.1590
289	PARATHYROID PROCEDURES	0.9573
290	THYROID PROCEDURES	0.8862
291	THYROGLOSSAL PROCEDURES	0.5964
292	OTHER ENDOCRINE, NUTRIT & METAB O.R. PROC W CC	2.6892
293	OTHER ENDOCRINE, NUTRIT & METAB O.R. PROC W/O CC	1.3059
294	DIABETES AGE >35	0.7608
295	DIABETES AGE 0-35	0.7457
296	NUTRITIONAL & MISC METABOLIC DISORDERS AGE >17 W CC	0.8615
297	NUTRITIONAL & MISC METABOLIC DISORDERS AGE >17 W/O CC	0.5047
298	NUTRITIONAL & MISC METABOLIC DISORDERS AGE 0-17	0.4155
299	INBORN ERRORS OF METABOLISM	0.9223
300	ENDOCRINE DISORDERS W CC	1.1243
301	ENDOCRINE DISORDERS W/O CC	0.6078
302	KIDNEY TRANSPLANT	3.3278
303	KIDNEY,URETER & MAJOR BLADDER PROCEDURES FOR NEOPLASM	2.4884
304	KIDNEY,URETER & MAJOR BLADDER PROC FOR NON-NEOPL W CC	2.4618
305	KIDNEY,URETER & MAJOR BLADDER PROC FOR NON-NEOPL W/O CC	1.1502
306	PROSTATECTOMY W CC	1.2988
307	PROSTATECTOMY W/O CC	0.6050
308	MINOR BLADDER PROCEDURES W CC	1.6896

Appendix 2

DRG Weights (cont.)

DRG	DRG Name	Weight
309	MINOR BLADDER PROCEDURES W/O CC	0.8936
310	TRANSURETHRAL PROCEDURES W CC	1.1366
311	TRANSURETHRAL PROCEDURES W/O CC	0.5957
312	URETHRAL PROCEDURES, AGE >17 W CC	1.0782
313	URETHRAL PROCEDURES, AGE >17 W/O CC	0.6584
314	URETHRAL PROCEDURES, AGE 0-17	0.4944
315	OTHER KIDNEY & URINARY TRACT O.R. PROCEDURES	2.1550
316	RENAL FAILURE	1.3745
317	ADMIT FOR RENAL DIALYSIS	0.6130
318	KIDNEY & URINARY TRACT NEOPLASMS W CC	1.1723
319	KIDNEY & URINARY TRACT NEOPLASMS W/O CC	0.5852
320	KIDNEY & URINARY TRACT INFECTIONS AGE >17 W CC	0.8593
321	KIDNEY & URINARY TRACT INFECTIONS AGE >17 W/O CC	0.5560
322	KIDNEY & URINARY TRACT INFECTIONS AGE 0-17	0.5267
323	URINARY STONES W CC, &/OR ESW LITHOTRIPSY	0.7970
324	URINARY STONES W/O CC	0.4422
325	KIDNEY & URINARY TRACT SIGNS & SYMPTOMS AGE >17 W CC	0.6336
326	KIDNEY & URINARY TRACT SIGNS & SYMPTOMS AGE >17 W/O CC	0.4120
327	KIDNEY & URINARY TRACT SIGNS & SYMPTOMS AGE 0-17	0.3697
328	URETHRAL STRICTURE AGE >17 W CC	0.7268
329	URETHRAL STRICTURE AGE >17 W/O CC	0.4458
330	URETHRAL STRICTURE AGE 0-17	0.3185
331	OTHER KIDNEY & URINARY TRACT DIAGNOSES AGE >17 W CC	1.0640
332	OTHER KIDNEY & URINARY TRACT DIAGNOSES AGE >17 W/O CC	0.6056
333	OTHER KIDNEY & URINARY TRACT DIAGNOSES AGE 0-17	0.7907
334	MAJOR MALE PELVIC PROCEDURES W CC	1.5177
335	MAJOR MALE PELVIC PROCEDURES W/O CC	1.1047
336	TRANSURETHRAL PROSTATECTOMY W CC	0.8630
337	TRANSURETHRAL PROSTATECTOMY W/O CC	0.5861
338	TESTES PROCEDURES, FOR MALIGNANCY	1.2191

Appendix 2

DRG Weights (cont.)

DRG	DRG Name	Weight
339	TESTES PROCEDURES, NON-MALIGNANCY AGE >17	1.1555
340	TESTES PROCEDURES, NON-MALIGNANCY AGE 0-17	0.2830
341	PENIS PROCEDURES	1.1306
342	CIRCUMCISION AGE >17	0.7852
343	CIRCUMCISION AGE 0-17	0.1538
344	OTHER MALE REPRODUCTIVE SYSTEM O.R. PROCEDURES FOR MALIGNANCY	1.1741
345	OTHER MALE REPRODUCTIVE SYSTEM O.R. PROC EXCEPT FOR MALIGNANCY	0.9149
346	MALIGNANCY, MALE REPRODUCTIVE SYSTEM, W CC	1.0304
347	MALIGNANCY, MALE REPRODUCTIVE SYSTEM, W/O CC	0.5660
348	BENIGN PROSTATIC HYPERTROPHY W CC	0.6998
349	BENIGN PROSTATIC HYPERTROPHY W/O CC	0.4128
350	INFLAMMATION OF THE MALE REPRODUCTIVE SYSTEM	0.7164
351	STERILIZATION, MALE	0.2360
352	OTHER MALE REPRODUCTIVE SYSTEM DIAGNOSES	0.6868
353	PELVIC EVISCERATION, RADICAL HYSTERECTOMY & RADICAL VULVECTOMY	1.8493
354	UTERINE,ADNEXA PROC FOR NON-OVARIAN/ADNEXAL MALIG W CC	1.5317
355	UTERINE,ADNEXA PROC FOR NON-OVARIAN/ADNEXAL MALIG W/O CC	0.9033
356	FEMALE REPRODUCTIVE SYSTEM RECONSTRUCTIVE PROCEDURES	0.7440
357	UTERINE & ADNEXA PROC FOR OVARIAN OR ADNEXAL MALIGNANCY	2.4380
358	UTERINE & ADNEXA PROC FOR NON-MALIGNANCY W CC	1.1902
359	UTERINE & ADNEXA PROC FOR NON-MALIGNANCY W/O CC	0.8165
360	VAGINA, CERVIX & VULVA PROCEDURES	0.8520
361	LAPAROSCOPY & INCISIONAL TUBAL INTERRUPTION	1.0964
362	ENDOSCOPIC TUBAL INTERRUPTION	0.3017
363	D&C, CONIZATION & RADIO-IMPLANT, FOR MALIGNANCY	0.8158
364	D&C, CONIZATION EXCEPT FOR MALIGNANCY	0.8170
365	OTHER FEMALE REPRODUCTIVE SYSTEM O.R. PROCEDURES	2.0008
366	MALIGNANCY, FEMALE REPRODUCTIVE SYSTEM W CC	1.2699

Appendix 2

DRG Weights (cont.)

DRG	DRG Name	Weight
367	MALIGNANCY, FEMALE REPRODUCTIVE SYSTEM W/O CC	0.5767
368	INFECTIONS, FEMALE REPRODUCTIVE SYSTEM	1.1355
369	MENSTRUAL & OTHER FEMALE REPRODUCTIVE SYSTEM DISORDERS	0.5581
370	CESAREAN SECTION W CC	1.0572
371	CESAREAN SECTION W/O CC	0.6845
372	VAGINAL DELIVERY W COMPLICATING DIAGNOSES	0.5550
373	VAGINAL DELIVERY W/O COMPLICATING DIAGNOSES	0.3774
374	VAGINAL DELIVERY W STERILIZATION &/OR D&C	0.6835
375	VAGINAL DELIVERY W O.R. PROC EXCEPT STERIL &/OR D&C	0.5759
376	POSTPARTUM & POST ABORTION DIAGNOSES W/O O.R. PROCEDURE	0.4963
377	POSTPARTUM & POST ABORTION DIAGNOSES W O.R. PROCEDURE	1.6892
378	ECTOPIC PREGNANCY	0.8017
379	THREATENED ABORTION	0.4521
380	ABORTION W/O D&C	0.4201
381	ABORTION W D&C, ASPIRATION CURETTAGE OR HYSTEROTOMY	0.6628
382	FALSE LABOR	0.1599
383	OTHER ANTEPARTUM DIAGNOSES W MEDICAL COMPLICATIONS	0.4915
384	OTHER ANTEPARTUM DIAGNOSES W/O MEDICAL COMPLICATIONS	0.3626
385	NEONATES, DIED OR TRANSFERRED TO ANOTHER ACUTE CARE FACILITY	1.3743
386	EXTREME IMMATURITY OR RESPIRATORY DISTRESS SYNDROME, NEONATE	4.5319
387	PREMATURITY W MAJOR PROBLEMS	3.0952
388	PREMATURITY W/O MAJOR PROBLEMS	1.8676
389	FULL TERM NEONATE W MAJOR PROBLEMS	3.1794
390	NEONATE W OTHER SIGNIFICANT PROBLEMS	1.1253
391	NORMAL NEWBORN	0.1524
392	SPLENECTOMY AGE >17	3.3892
393	SPLENECTOMY AGE 0-17	1.3462
394	OTHER O.R. PROCEDURES OF THE BLOOD AND BLOOD FORMING	1.8231

Appendix 2

DRG Weights (cont.)

DRG	DRG Name	Weight
	ORGANS	
395	RED BLOOD CELL DISORDERS AGE >17	0.8192
396	RED BLOOD CELL DISORDERS AGE 0-17	1.0407
397	COAGULATION DISORDERS	1.2671
398	RETICULOENDOTHELIAL & IMMUNITY DISORDERS W CC	1.3082
399	RETICULOENDOTHELIAL & IMMUNITY DISORDERS W/O CC	0.6675
400	LYMPHOMA & LEUKEMIA W MAJOR O.R. PROCEDURE	2.9346
401	LYMPHOMA & NON-ACUTE LEUKEMIA W OTHER O.R. PROC W CC	2.9905
402	LYMPHOMA & NON-ACUTE LEUKEMIA W OTHER O.R. PROC W/O CC	1.1594
403	LYMPHOMA & NON-ACUTE LEUKEMIA W CC	1.8579
404	LYMPHOMA & NON-ACUTE LEUKEMIA W/O CC	0.8718
405	ACUTE LEUKEMIA W/O MAJOR O.R. PROCEDURE AGE 0-17	1.9086
406	MYELOPROLIF DISORD OR POORLY DIFF NEOPL W MAJ O.R.PROC W CC	2.9939
407	MYELOPROLIF DISORD OR POORLY DIFF NEOPL W MAJ O.R.PROC W/O CC	1.2426
408	MYELOPROLIF DISORD OR POORLY DIFF NEOPL W OTHER O.R.PROC	2.2144
409	RADIOTHERAPY	1.1575
410	CHEMOTHERAPY W/O ACUTE LEUKEMIA AS SECONDARY DIAGNOSIS	0.9991
411	HISTORY OF MALIGNANCY W/O ENDOSCOPY	0.4481
412	HISTORY OF MALIGNANCY W ENDOSCOPY	0.5958
413	OTHER MYELOPROLIF DIS OR POORLY DIFF NEOPL DIAG W CC	1.3894
414	OTHER MYELOPROLIF DIS OR POORLY DIFF NEOPL DIAG W/O CC	0.7418
415	O.R. PROCEDURE FOR INFECTIOUS & PARASITIC DISEASES	3.9067
416	SEPTICEMIA AGE >17	1.6226
417	SEPTICEMIA AGE 0-17	0.8915
418	POSTOPERATIVE & POST-TRAUMATIC INFECTIONS	1.0493
419	FEVER OF UNKNOWN ORIGIN AGE >17 W CC	0.8618
420	FEVER OF UNKNOWN ORIGIN AGE >17 W/O CC	0.6112
421	VIRAL ILLNESS AGE >17	0.6640

Appendix 2

DRG Weights (cont.)

DRG	DRG Name	Weight
422	VIRAL ILLNESS & FEVER OF UNKNOWN ORIGIN AGE 0-17	0.4757
423	OTHER INFECTIOUS & PARASITIC DISEASES DIAGNOSES	1.8365
424	O.R. PROCEDURE W PRINCIPAL DIAGNOSES OF MENTAL ILLNESS	2.4518
425	ACUTE ADJUSTMENT REACTION & PSYCHOSOCIAL DYSFUNCTION	0.6789
426	DEPRESSIVE NEUROSES	0.5261
427	NEUROSES EXCEPT DEPRESSIVE	0.5348
428	DISORDERS OF PERSONALITY & IMPULSE CONTROL	0.7242
429	ORGANIC DISTURBANCES & MENTAL RETARDATION	0.8367
430	PSYCHOSES	0.7676
431	CHILDHOOD MENTAL DISORDERS	0.6416
432	OTHER MENTAL DISORDER DIAGNOSES	0.7100
433	ALCOHOL/DRUG ABUSE OR DEPENDENCE, LEFT AMA	0.2888
434	NO LONGER VALID	0.0000
435	NO LONGER VALID	0.0000
436	NO LONGER VALID	0.0000
437	NO LONGER VALID	0.0000
438	NO LONGER VALID	0.0000
439	SKIN GRAFTS FOR INJURIES	1.9332
440	WOUND DEBRIDEMENTS FOR INJURIES	2.0806
441	HAND PROCEDURES FOR INJURIES	0.9295
442	OTHER O.R. PROCEDURES FOR INJURIES W CC	2.5304
443	OTHER O.R. PROCEDURES FOR INJURIES W/O CC	0.9920
444	TRAUMATIC INJURY AGE >17 W CC	0.7277
445	TRAUMATIC INJURY AGE >17 W/O CC	0.4716
446	TRAUMATIC INJURY AGE 0-17	0.2959
447	ALLERGIC REACTIONS AGE >17	0.4825
448	ALLERGIC REACTIONS AGE 0-17	0.0973
449	POISONING & TOXIC EFFECTS OF DRUGS AGE >17 W CC	0.8309
450	POISONING & TOXIC EFFECTS OF DRUGS AGE >17 W/O CC	0.4139
451	POISONING & TOXIC EFFECTS OF DRUGS AGE 0-17	0.2627

Appendix 2

DRG Weights (cont.)

DRG	DRG Name	Weight
452	COMPLICATIONS OF TREATMENT W CC	1.0122
453	COMPLICATIONS OF TREATMENT W/O CC	0.4980
454	OTHER INJURY, POISONING & TOXIC EFFECT DIAG W CC	0.8692
455	OTHER INJURY, POISONING & TOXIC EFFECT DIAG W/O CC	0.4630
456	NO LONGER VALID	0.0000
457	NO LONGER VALID	0.0000
458	NO LONGER VALID	0.0000
459	NO LONGER VALID	0.0000
460	NO LONGER VALID	0.0000
461	O.R. PROC W DIAGNOSES OF OTHER CONTACT W HEALTH SERVICES	1.1963
462	REHABILITATION	1.2125
463	SIGNS & SYMPTOMS W CC	0.6800
464	SIGNS & SYMPTOMS W/O CC	0.4628
465	AFTERCARE W HISTORY OF MALIGNANCY AS SECONDARY DIAGNOSIS	0.5445
466	AFTERCARE W/O HISTORY OF MALIGNANCY AS SECONDARY DIAGNOSIS	0.6416
467	OTHER FACTORS INFLUENCING HEALTH STATUS	0.4585
468	EXTENSIVE O.R. PROCEDURE UNRELATED TO PRINCIPAL DIAGNOSIS	3.8756
469	PRINCIPAL DIAGNOSIS INVALID AS DISCHARGE DIAGNOSIS	0.0000
470	UNGROUPABLE	0.0000
471	BILATERAL OR MULTIPLE MAJOR JOINT PROCS OF LOWER EXTREMITY	3.0067
472	NO LONGER VALID	0.0000
473	ACUTE LEUKEMIA W/O MAJOR O.R. PROCEDURE AGE >17	3.9324
474	NO LONGER VALID	0.0000
475	RESPIRATORY SYSTEM DIAGNOSIS WITH VENTILATOR SUPPORT	3.9253
476	PROSTATIC O.R. PROCEDURE UNRELATED TO PRINCIPAL DIAGNOSIS	2.2915
477	NON-EXTENSIVE O.R. PROCEDURE UNRELATED TO PRINCIPAL DIAGNOSIS	1.9568

Appendix 2

DRG Weights (cont.)

DRG	DRG Name	Weight
478	OTHER VASCULAR PROCEDURES W CC	2.4161
479	OTHER VASCULAR PROCEDURES W/O CC	1.3900
480	LIVER TRANSPLANT	10.9812
481	BONE MARROW TRANSPLANT	8.0438
482	TRACHEOSTOMY FOR FACE,MOUTH & NECK DIAGNOSES	3.8583
483	TRACHEOSTOMY EXCEPT FOR FACE,MOUTH & NECK DIAGNOSES	15.4629
484	CRANIOTOMY FOR MULTIPLE SIGNIFICANT TRAUMA	5.2963
485	LIMB REATTACHMENT, HIP AND FEMUR PROC FOR MULTIPLE SIGNIFICANT TRA	3.1724
486	OTHER O.R. PROCEDURES FOR MULTIPLE SIGNIFICANT TRAUMA	5.2888
487	OTHER MULTIPLE SIGNIFICANT TRAUMA	1.9585
488	HIV W EXTENSIVE O.R. PROCEDURE	5.1965
489	HIV W MAJOR RELATED CONDITION	1.8948
490	HIV W OR W/O OTHER RELATED CONDITION	1.0584
491	MAJOR JOINT & LIMB REATTACHMENT PROCEDURES OF UPPER EXTREMITY	1.6353
492	CHEMOTHERAPY W ACUTE LEUKEMIA AS SECONDARY DIAGNOSIS	4.8886
493	LAPAROSCOPIC CHOLECYSTECTOMY W/O C.D.E. W CC	1.8411
494	LAPAROSCOPIC CHOLECYSTECTOMY W/O C.D.E. W/O CC	0.9754
495	LUNG TRANSPLANT	8.8252
496	COMBINED ANTERIOR/POSTERIOR SPINAL FUSION	5.7281
497	SPINAL FUSION EXCEPT CERVICAL W CC	3.2324
498	SPINAL FUSION EXCEPT CERVICAL W/O CC	2.3026
499	BACK & NECK PROCEDURES EXCEPT SPINAL FUSION W CC	1.4507
500	BACK & NECK PROCEDURES EXCEPT SPINAL FUSION W/O CC	0.9385
501	KNEE PROCEDURES W PDX OF INFECTION W CC	2.7485
502	KNEE PROCEDURES W PDX OF INFECTION W/O CC	1.5544
503	KNEE PROCEDURES W/O PDX OF INFECTION	1.2291
504	EXTENSIVE 3RD DEGREE BURNS W SKIN GRAFT	14.1729
505	EXTENSIVE 3RD DEGREE BURNS W/O SKIN GRAFT	1.4994
506	FULL THICKNESS BURN W SKIN GRAFT OR INHAL INJ W CC OR SIG	4.9233

Appendix 2

DRG Weights (cont.)

DRG	DRG Name	Weight
	TRAUMA	
507	FULL THICKNESS BURN W SKIN GRFT OR INHAL INJ W/O CC OR SIG TRAUMA	1.8583
508	FULL THICKNESS BURN W/O SKIN GRFT OR INHAL INJ W CC OR SIG TRAUMA	1.2967
509	FULL THICKNESS BURN W/O SKIN GRFT OR INH INJ W/O CC OR SIG TRAUMA	0.7265
510	NON-EXTENSIVE BURNS W CC OR SIGNIFICANT TRAUMA	1.3681
511	NON-EXTENSIVE BURNS W/O CC OR SIGNIFICANT TRAUMA	0.7656
512	SIMULTANEOUS PANCREAS/KIDNEY TRANSPLANT	5.7813
513	PANCREAS TRANSPLANT	5.8400
514	CARDIAC DEFIBRILLATOR IMPLANT W CARDIAC CATH	6.3663
515	CARDIAC DEFIBRILLATOR IMPLANT W/O CARDIAC CATH	4.9905
516	PERCUTANEOUS CARDIOVASC PROC W AMI	2.7475
517	PERC CARDIO PROC W CORONARY ARTERY STENT W/O AMI	2.1379
518	PERC CARDIO PROC W/O CORONARY ARTERY STENT OR AMI	1.6989
519	CERVICAL SPINAL FUSION W CC	2.3249
520	CERVICAL SPINAL FUSION W/O CC	1.4195
521	ALCOHOL/DRUG ABUSE OR DEPENDENCE W CC	0.7355
522	ALC/DRUG ABUSE OR DEPEND W REHABILITATION THERAPY W/O CC	0.6249
523	ALC/DRUG ABUSE OR DEPEND W/O REHABILITATION THERAPY W/O CC	0.3997

Appendix 3

DISCHARGE SUMMARY #1

PATIENT NAME:
ACCOUNT #:
MED REC #:
SEX/AGE: **Female/78**
STATUS/LOC:
DEPT/RT:

ADMISSION DATE: 09/29/01
DISCHARGE DATE: 10/22/01
ATTENDING PHYSICIAN:

HISTORY OF PRESENT ILLNESS: This 78-year-old female was brought in from a nursing home with multiple decubiti, dehydration, respiratory distress, congestion, and not responding to antibiotic as a nursing home patient. The patient had suffered a stroke and has been in contracture with PEG feeding, aphasic and had multiple decubiti, as well as vascular disease with gangrene of her fingers, mostly on the right hand and elbow, contracture left with decubiti.

ALLERGIES: The patient has no known drug allergies.

HOSPITAL COURSE: All the cultures were done, IV hydration was started, her hypotension was corrected, and the patient was given IV antibiotics and IV hydration and PEG feeding was started. Pain management was done, and the patient continued to show some improvement, but later on her condition became more unstable, and she has not been clearing up her pneumonia. She kept on getting recurrent pneumonia, as well as UTI not clearing up. It became a yeast infection. Her family agreed for DNR and comfort case measures only.

DISCHARGE DIAGNOSES: Septic shock, Parkinson's disease, post-CVA dehydration, multiple decubiti, aspiration pneumonia, urinary tract infection and pain management, renal insufficiency, anemia and dehydration.

MEDICATIONS ON DISCHARGE: Morphine elixir 15 mg per 5 cc q. 4h. p.r.n. pain, Duragesic patch 75 mcg q. 72h., Tylenol elixir by G-tube or 650 mg suppository q.i.d. for pain and temperature over 100. The patient will also continue to get Colace 200 mg by PEG, Sinemet 25/250 by PEG t.i.d., zinc 220 mg by PEG q.d., vitamin C 500 mg by

Appendix 3

DISCHARGE SUMMARY #1 (cont.)

PEG q.d., Catapres 0.1 mg by PEG b.i.d. (hold if systolic blood pressure is 120 or lower, diastolic blood pressure 90 or lower), ProMod two scoops by G-tube t.i.d., Reglan 10 mg PEG q.i.d.

DISCHARGE INSTRUCTIONS: Her dressing order has been written. She will be also on Humibid 600 mg by PEG b.i.d. She will require frequent suctioning, oxygen via nasal cannula or by mask, whichever way the patient is comfortable. Her PEG feeding will be ____ feeding with Iso source or equivalent 40 cc/hour with free water. Her wound dressing is enclosed. Her worst wounds are in the sacral and in the gluteal areas. The rest of them are drying and can get a little more open air, but her sacral decubitus should be cleaned with saline and apply Accuzyme q.d.

Also to the right hip decubitus, clean with saline and apply Accuzyme. PEG site: Clean with normal saline and apply Bactroban q. shift.

PRINCIPAL DIAGNOSIS:

____

SECONDARY DIAGNOSES:

____

Appendix 3

DISCHARGE SUMMARY #2

PATIENT NAME:
ACCOUNT #:
MED REC #:
SEX/AGE:
STATUS/LOC:
DEPT/RT:

ADMISSION DATE: 10/15/01
DISCHARGE DATE: 10/18/01
ATTENDING PHYSICIAN:

HISTORY OF PRESENT ILLNESS: Multiple falls over the last 4 months with recurrent fractures, particularly of the pelvis, wrist and ribs. The patient keeps on falling despite one-to-one caregiver at home. The patient has been becoming a little bit more confused lately. She was admitted to the emergency room where she had a broken cast of the right wrist area. The patient was mildly dehydrated on admission and started on IV fluids.

PAST MEDICAL HISTORY: Hypertension, congestive heart failure, anemia, cardiomyopathy, depression.

HOSPITAL COURSE: During the hospital course the patient was seen by the neurologist, who felt that she may have normal pressure hydrocephalus vs. a new stroke or spinal pathology. CAT scan of the brain showed no acute changes. An MRI of the brain showed ?? and severe atrophy. Her MRI of the thoracic spine did not show any acute pathology. The patient was arranged to have physical therapy and occupational therapy. She and her daughter have been explained that she needs to continue with these treatments to prevent any falls and/or fractures.

Of importance, he lab work shows a hemoglobin and hematocrit of 9.8 and 29.4 with a white count of 3900. Her sodium was 140, potassium 3.4, blood sugar normal, BUN 25 and creatinine has been within normal limits. She ruled out for an MI. Her thyroid function tests were within normal limits. Urinalysis was normal.

Appendix 3

DISCHARGE SUMMARY #2 (cont.)

EKG shows normal sinus rhythm with first-degree AV block and non-specific ST-T changes.

Her x-rays show some broken ribs on the right side.

The patient is being transferred to a nursing home with a diagnosis of syncopal episode, dementia, cardiomyopathy, hypertension and hypothyroidism.

We appreciate Dr. ________, the consultation, who also agrees with the present treatment and transferring to the nursing home.

PRINCIPAL DIAGNOSIS:

____

SECONDARY DIAGNOSES:

____

Appendix 3

DISCHARGE SUMMARY #3

PATIENT NAME:
ACCOUNT #:
MED REC #:
SEX/AGE:
STATUS/LOC:
DEPT/RT:

ADMISSION DATE: 10/09/01
DISCHARGE DATE: 10/15/01
ATTENDING PHYSICIAN:

DISCHARGE DIAGNOSES: Lower gastrointestinal bleed, most likely secondary to diverticulosis. Hypothyroidism. Osteoporosis.

HOSPITAL COURSE: The patient has a history of diverticular bleed 10 years ago and 4 years ago at hospital. He was hospitalized with bright red blood and dark red blood per rectum. An upper endoscopy at that time revealed gastritis. Colonoscopy at that time revealed marked diverticulosis and possible right AVM. There was no active bleeding.

He came into the hospital with two days of bright red blood and dark red blood per rectum, without hematemesis or melena. He was mildly orthostatic on admission. He was transfused 2 units of packed red blood cells. His admission hematocrit was 28.1. His hematocrit was only 27.3 after 2 units and he was given a third unit with a rise to 30.4. However, on 10/11/01, two days after his admission, he again bled and his hematocrit dropped to 26.9. He was transferred to the step-down ICU and underwent a colonoscopy on 10/12/01 which revealed marked diverticulosis without evidence of active bleeding. He was advanced to a regular diet. He received a total of 7 units of packed red blood cells. His hematocrit was stable at approximately 28 to 30. He feels well now. He was evaluated by physical therapy who felt that he was slightly unstable on walking and could benefit from a cane. He was evaluated by social work for possible discharge to ________________ for continued physical therapy and rehabilitation.

At the time of discharge, white count is 4.3, hematocrit 28.4, platelet count 100. BUN is 12, creatinine 1.0.

Appendix 3

DISCHARGE SUMMARY #3 (cont.)

DISCHARGE MEDICATIONS: Synthroid 0.1 mg q.day, Actonel and pituitary medicine once per week.

DISCHARGE INSTRUCTIONS: The patient can follow-up as needed. He is to call my office or come to the emergency room if he has further bleeding.

PRINCIPAL DIAGNOSIS:

SECONDARY DIAGNOSES:

Appendix 3

DISCHARGE SUMMARY #4

PATIENT NAME:
ACCOUNT #:
MED REC #:
SEX/AGE:
STATUS/LOC:
DEPT/RT:

ADMISSION DATE: 10/18/01
DISCHARGE DATE: 10/23/01
ATTENDING PHYSICIAN:

DISCHARGE DIAGNOSES:
Intractable low back pain, multifactorial.
Osteoarthritis and possible spinal stenosis of the lumbar back.
Urinary tract infection with possible urosepsis.
Type 2 diabetes mellitus.
Hypertension.
Glaucoma.
History of depression.
History of renal cell carcinoma, status post previous nephrectomy.
Previous stroke in the past.
Mild dementia.

DISCHARGE INSTRUCTIONS:
The patient is being discharged to a nursing home for ongoing care.
Daily physical therapy and occupational therapy.
An 1800-calorie, 3-gram sodium diet.

DISCHARGE MEDICATIONS:
Ceftin 250 mg p.o. b.i.d. for 3 days.
Captopril 6.25 mg p.o. t.i.d.
Darvocet one to two tablets p.o. t.i.d. p.r.n.
Aspirin 81 mg q.d.
Atenolol 10 mg q.d.
BuSpar 10 mg p.o. q.d.

Appendix 3

DISCHARGE SUMMARY #4 (cont.)

Diabenase 125 mg p.o. q.d.
Detrol 2 mg p.o. q.d.
Colace 100 mg p.o. b.i.d.

BRIEF HISTORY: Patient is an 83-year-old gentleman from assisted living who presents with severe low back pain. For complete history and physical please see admitting history and physical.

DATA:
CT scan of the abdomen and pelvis on admission showed previous right nephrectomy. No evidence of abdominal aortic aneurysm. There was a cholelithiasis but no evidence of a cholecystitis.
X-rays of the lumbosacral spine showed evidence of osteoarthritis.
Chest x-ray was clear.

HOSPITAL COURSE: The patient was admitted to a regular medical bed. He had been evaluated in the emergency department including a CT scan of the abdomen and pelvis and an abdominal ultrasound that was unremarkable. A urinalysis did show evidence of a urinary tract infection and the patient was started on intravenous antibiotics. He was also started on intravenous fluids and oral pain medication. Plain films of the back were obtained which did show evidence of osteoarthritis.

The patient received daily physical therapy. Over the next few days, his symptoms did improve and his pain was controlled with oral pain medications. He was quite weak, however, and required maximal assistance for ambulating. After a few days of physical therapy, he was ambulating 30 feet with a walker and with assistance. His mental status was essentially at baseline.

By the date of discharge, the patient was medically stable. He is going to be going to a local nursing home for ongoing care at this time.

PRINCIPAL DIAGNOSIS:

____

SECONDARY DIAGNOSES:

____

Appendix 3

DISCHARGE SUMMARY #5

PATIENT NAME:
ACCOUNT #:
MED REC #:
SEX/AGE:
STATUS/LOC:
DEPT/RT:

ADMISSION DATE: 10/24/01
DISCHARGE DATE: 10/30/01
ATTENDING PHYSICIAN:

DISCHARGE DIAGNOSES:
Right hip fracture status post open reduction, internal fixation by Dr. __________ on 10/19/01.
Osteoporosis.
Type II diabetes mellitus.
Hypertension.
History of congestive heart failure.
History of coronary artery disease status coronary artery bypass grafting.

DISCHARGE INSTRUCTIONS:
The patient is being discharged to home.
She has been instructed to follow up with her primary care physician next week.
She has been instructed that she needs to have a protime and INR checked weekly while she is on Coumadin.

DISCHARGE MEDICATIONS:
Atenolol 50 mg daily.
Diovan 160 mg daily.
Glyburide 5 mg po bid.
Lisinopril 20 mg po bid.
Coumadin 2.5 mg one daily.
Fosamax 70 mg po qAM.
Lasix 40 mg po qAM.
Glucophage 850 mg po bid.

Appendix 3

DISCHARGE SUMMARY #5 (cont.)

Calcium 500 mg with vitamin D 200 units one tablet three times daily.
Vicodin 1-2 tablets po q4h PRN.

REHABILITATION COURSE: The patient was admitted for rehabilitation after having undergone open reduction, internal fixation of a right hip fracture a few days earlier in the hospital. She received daily physical therapy and occupational therapy. Her blood pressure was slightly elevated, but improved when we got her back on a regular antihypertensive regimen. Her blood sugars remained well controlled. There were no complications during her rehabilitation stay. She progressed well with physical therapy and is going home at this time. She was maintained on Coumadin for deep venous thrombosis prophylaxis.

PRINCIPAL DIAGNOSIS:

____

SECONDARY DIAGNOSES:

____

Appendix 3

DISCHARGE SUMMARY #6

PATIENT NAME:
ACCOUNT #:
MED REC #:
SEX/AGE:
STATUS/LOC:
DEPT/RT:

ADMISSION DATE:
DISCHARGE DATE:
ATTENDING PHYSICIAN:

HISTORY OF PRESENT ILLNESS: This is a 33-year-old female with a well known history of ulcerative colitis. The patient was admitted to the hospital with abdominal pain and chest pain radiating to her neck and right shoulder. Noted to have a hematocrit of 20 and hemoglobin of 6. The patient had a fever of 102, chills and mild diarrhea. No mucus but some blood in the stool. Her bowel movements had been about two a day for the last few weeks. The patient went for a second opinion the day of admission. She will wait for therapy as an outpatient at ______________ Hospital, where she will go on November 7th.

HOSPITAL COURSE: The patient was admitted, blood cultures were obtained, and all of them were within the normal limits. The initial chest x-ray was negative. The second chest x-ray showed a left lower lobe infiltrate. By that time, the patient was already on Levaquin 500 IV and she had already received two doses. We did a CT of the thorax to rule out pulmonary embolism and a pericardial effusion, and that was ruled out in the beginning. Her oxygenation has been normal. The patient received two units of PRBCs on this admission and she felt quite improved. Her chest pain improved. Her abdominal pain was none. At this time, her white count was normal and her hematocrit rose to 11.3 and 34. The patient was seen kindly in consultation by her gastroenterologist, who put her on IV steroids, requested an abdominal sonogram which was within normal limits, and a CT scan of the abdomen and pelvis was negative. She is going to go home on Levaquin 500 mg IV, Prednisone 30 mg p.o., Protonix 40 b.i.d. She will continue with her Aggrenox, and she will be on Cortenemas once a day and Asacol.

Appendix 3

DISCHARGE SUMMARY #6 (cont.)

FINAL DIAGNOSES:

Pneumonia, left lower lobe infiltrate.
Sepsis.
Anemia, acute.
Gastrointestinal bleeding, lower from ulcerative colitis, aggressive.
Status post-cerebrovascular accident in August 2001.

PLAN: The patient will be followed as an outpatient and get an H&H in 48 hours in my office and then she will be seen in three days.

PRINCIPAL DIAGNOSIS:

____

SECONDARY DIAGNOSES:

____

Appendix 3

DISCHARGE SUMMARY #7

PATIENT NAME:
ACCOUNT #:
MED REC #:
SEX/AGE: Male/93
STATUS/LOC:
DEPT/RT:

ADMISSION DATE: 10/14/01
DISCHARGE DATE:
ATTENDING PHYSICIAN:

DISCHARGE DIAGNOSES:
Change in mental status.
Hyponatremia.
Status post-obstructive uropathy.
History of chronic atrial fibrillation.
History of hypertension.
History of asthma.
History of glaucoma.
History of benign prostatic hypertrophy.
History of scoliosis.
History of cerebrovascular accident.
History of anemia.

HISTORY OF PRESENT ILLNESS: Please see history and physical on admission for details. The patient is a 93-year-old-man brought to the hospital after sustaining a fall in his assisted living apartment. The patient was not able to give any history on admission and was confused. The patient was worked up in the emergency room with x-rays, CT scans and lab data.

HOSPITAL COURSE: The patient was admitted to the medical floor and was continued on IV antibiotics, and a Foley catheter was placed. The patient was seen in consultation, neurology, and by nephrology. The patient underwent a workup by urology and nephrology, with improvement in his mental status. The patient underwent EEG per

Appendix 3

DISCHARGE SUMMARY #7 (cont.)

neurology, and it was felt by neurology that ________________ was most likely metabolic in etiology.

The patient's mental status did improve, with improvement in his serum sodium. The patient also underwent nutrition evaluation. The patient was also noted to be orthostatic. The patient was continued on Coumadin with therapeutic INR. The patient was stable for transfer to home. The patient was cleared by nephrology and neurology for transfer.

MEDICATIONS ON DISCHARGE: Fluticasone 110 mcg 2 puffs cystoscope, Nitro-Dur 0.4 mg/hour q.d. on a.m. and on p.m., lisinopril 20 mg. p.o. q.d., doxazosin 4 mg p.o. q.d., Datril, Atrovent and Combivent inhaler 4 puffs q.i.d., atenolol 6.25 mg p.o. q.d., Coumadin 2.5 mg p.o. q.d., Flomax 0.8 mg p.o. q.d. after lunch.

DISCHARGE INSTRUCTIONS: The patient needs to have his PT/INR monitored while on Coumadin and also have a DMP monitored. One can of Boost or equivalent p.o. b.i.d.

PRINCIPAL DIAGNOSIS:

____

SECONDARY DIAGNOSES:

____

Appendix 3

DISCHARGE SUMMARY #8

PATIENT NAME:
ACCOUNT #:
MED REC #:
SEX/AGE:
STATUS/LOC:
DEPT/RT:

ADMISSION DATE:
DISCHARGE DATE:
ATTENDING PHYSICIAN:

PROBLEMS: Patient admitted with diarrhea and dehydration. History of T4 colon cancer.

PERTINENT LABORATORY DATA: Patient with Clostridium difficile positive stool culture from 10/16/01.

HOSPITAL COURSE: Patient was admitted to hospital with diarrhea and dehydration. As per HPI she was receiving infusional 5-fluorouracil and radiation therapy concurrently. She also had significant mouth ulceration. Interestingly, her stool was positive for Clostridium difficile. The patient was managed with aggressive intravenous hydration and oral Flagyl with improvement. She also required electrolyte replacement on several occasions. By the time of discharge she was markedly improved. She did have some low grade temperatures which were presumed secondary to her Clostridium difficile infection.

DISPOSITION: She will be discharged to home and will follow up in our office within the next several days.

DISCHARGE MEDICATIONS:
Flagyl 500 tid.
Magic mouthwash.

When she returns to the office we will check a CBC, CMP +4.

PRINCIPAL DIAGNOSIS:

SECONDARY DIAGNOSES:

Related Products from HCPro

Books

Guide to Compliance Auditing: Applying OIG Techniques and Tools

With all the corporate compliance resources out there, why would you need this book, too?

The answer is simple: *Guide to Compliance Auditing: Applying OIG Techniques and Tools* is the only book of its kind that's written by an actual former compliance auditor with the inside scoop on how the OIG conducts its audits. This book provides compliance officers and internal auditors with the same principles and tried-and-true techniques that the DHHS OIG uses to conduct audits of the Medicare and Medicaid programs. teams and governing boards.

Not only does this book provide one-of-a-kind information, it makes the information easy to understand and put into action in your facility. With *Guide to Compliance Auditing: Applying OIG Techniques and Tools,* you'll:

- Learn how to plan a compliance audit
- Have ready-to-use standards working papers the OIG developed and uses
- Know how to write credible and convincing audit reports
- Follow easy, step-by-step audit programs for hot areas such as research and bad debts
- Understand why the OIG's audits are consistently successful, credible, and convincing
- Learn how to apply The Government Auditing Standards to your own compliance and monitoring program

Simply stated, with *Guide to Compliance Auditing: Applying OIG Techniques and Tools,* you'll have the knowledge and confidence to effectively and efficiently audit and monitor healthcare laws to maintain your compliance, and thus avoid the negative consequences of noncompliance.

Corporate Compliance Manual for Physician Practices

This manual will help you establish and manage an effective corporate compliance program. It is an easy-to-use, comprehensive, how-to guide to understanding the federal fraud and abuse regulations as they apply to medical practices. It includes sample policies and procedures that you can download from the Web and tailor to your own practice! With *Corporate Compliance Manual for Physician Practices,* you'll be able to

- Truly understand the OIG requirements, with the author's plain-English analysis and explanations
- Adapt the sample policies and procedures provided to fit your own compliance program
- Create your own compliance tools from the model forms included, such as compliance issue intake forms, compliance officer's job description, and E&M documentation and coding forms
- Understand Phase I of the new, final Stark II physician self-referral law
- Use the author's tips and strategies to design a corporate compliance program that fits your practice
- Prepare for OIG and CMS investigations
- Carry out effective internal compliance investigations
- Plus, it includes sample handouts and PowerPoint presentation slides that you can tailor to your own compliance education needs.

Corporate Compliance: Education and Training Programs

Many training directors and compliance officers have told us that they'd like to have a practical guide on how to design an effective corporate compliance training program. Not only is creating the content for such a program labor-intensive, but choosing and designing the most effective and appropriate training modes is difficult and time-consuming, too. That's why we're pleased to offer you *Corporate Compliance: Education and Training Programs.*

Written by former Inspector General Richard P. Kusserow and corporate compliance expert William R. O'Rourke, this guide provides all of the necessary guidelines and materials you'll need to meet the government's requirements for your corporate compliance training program. With it, you'll

- Learn about several teaching modes and be able to choose the most appropriate ones for your purposes and staff members
- Adapt the sample training schedules to suit your needs
- Use the book's authoritative training content in your own training program
- Tailor the sample scripts and materials to fit your training sessions
- Employ the tips and strategies that the authors offer to make your training program as effective as possible

You can use *Corporate Compliance: Education and Training Programs* for all training purposes, from orientation of new staff members to refresher sessions for your more experienced staff. It will save you countless hours you'd otherwise spend creating your own corporate compliance training materials. And because the authors have experience and expertise and provide authoritative and comprehensive content for your presentations, you won't have to worry about whether you're covering all you need to cover to meet the government's requirements.

Newsletters

Mammography Regulation Report

The FDA has recently stepped up its enforcement of the Mammography Quality Standards Act regulations, issuing hundreds of warning letters to first-time and repeat violators. *Mammography Regulation Report: Your Guide to a Successful FDA Inspection and Overall Federal Compliance* will help you meet the FDA's high-quality standards. Published monthly, *Mammography Regulation Report* is a new, 12-page newsletter focusing on the regulations that affect directors of mammography, directors of radiology, administrators, chief x-ray technologists, mammography supervisors and techs. Topics covered in *Mammography Regulation Report* include:

- Explanations of FDA regulations and advice on how to make compliance easier
- Reminders on staff, education, and licenses
- How to train new x-ray technologists to ensure they are committed to compliance from day one
- How to prepare for your annual FDA inspection
- Tips on improving mammography quality and interpretation
- Analysis of FDA warning letters
- Coding tips to ensure proper reimbursement
- Create phantom images
- Film expert advice on mammogram positioning and compression-two problem areas, according to FDA inspectors
- Advice from the FDA and American College of Radiology
- How to manage the paper trail
- Solutions for efficient record-keeping
- Updates on equipment

Corporate Compliance Officer

The government is stepping up EMTALA enforcement. Compliance with the final HIPAA privacy regulations will test the budget and resources of every healthcare provider. And now that you've finally got a handle on the anti-kickback statute, along comes Stark II—and a whole new set of headaches. As a compliance professional, your responsibilities have never loomed as large—and your need for information has never been greater. Let this monthly publication be your guide to establishing and maintaining an effective compliance program.